CARDIOLOGY RESEARCH AND CLINICAL DEVELOPMENTS

MITRAL VALVE DISEASE

DIAGNOSIS, TREATMENT AND FUTURE THERAPY

CARDIOLOGY RESEARCH AND CLINICAL DEVELOPMENTS

Additional books in this series can be found on Nova's website under the Series tab.

Additional e-books in this series can be found on Nova's website under the e-book tab.

CARDIOLOGY RESEARCH AND CLINICAL DEVELOPMENTS

MITRAL VALVE DISEASE

DIAGNOSIS, TREATMENT AND FUTURE THERAPY

RICHARD R. HEUSER
EDITOR

Nova Science Publishers, Inc.
New York

For permission to use material from this book please contact us:
Telephone 631-231-7269; Fax 631-231-8175
Web Site: http://www.novapublishers.com

Additional color graphics may be available in the e-book version of this book.

Library of Congress Cataloging-in-Publication Data

ISBN: 978-1-61942-309-1

Published by Nova Science Publishers, Inc. † New York

CONTENTS

PREFACE

This book discusses the different aspects of mitral regurgitation as well as diagnostic and imaging studies to evaluate the patients at risk. Treatment options for patients with mitral regurgitation are discussed including some of the new non-surgical treatments. Various medical devices and technologies have evolved recently making the traditional surgery not the only option in these patients. This book will be helpful to surgeons, cardiologists, as well as other clinicians and students interested in the diagnosis and treatment of mitral regurgitation.

Chapter 1 - Degenerative mitral valve (MV) disease is the most common form of organic non-ischemic MV regurgitation. Myxomatous degeneration commonly involves the annulus, the leaflets and the subvalvular apparatus. Three forms of degenerative mitral valve disease have been described based on the extent and degree of degenerative changes: Barlow's disease, Fibro-elastic deficiency and Forme Froste. Quantitative grading of mitral regurgitation is a powerful predictor of the clinical outcome of asymptomatic mitral regurgitation. The combination of symptoms and echocardiographic assessment (severity of regurgitation, left ventricular size and function, left atrial size and pulmonary artery systolic pressure) guides the timing of surgical intervention. MV replacement with either a biologic or mechanical prosthesis used to be the standard of care for surgical treatment of degenerative MV regurgitation. A variety of MV repair techniques have been developed with a success rate of 90% in expert hands at high volume centers. The choice of specific repair technique is based on the segmental analysis of the mitral valve preoperatively using Echocardiography and intra-operatively by direct visualization. The results of surgical treatment of degenerative mitral valve disease are dependent on the extent of the disease, technique used and the preoperative ventricular function. The authors review in this chapter the pathophysiology of degenerative mitral valve regurgitation, its natural history and echocardiographic assessment of mitral regurgitation caused by degenerative MV disease. This review discusses also different surgical techniques used to treat degenerative MV regurgitation and the results of these techniques supported by up to date review of the literature.

Chapter 2 - Ischemic mitral regurgitation (IMR) is present in 10%-20% of patients with Coronary Artery Disease (CAD) and is associated with a markedly worse prognosis and long-term patient survival in comparison with other types of mitral regurgitation. IMR can be classified into an acute type and a chronic type. Acute IMR occurs as a result of papillary muscle rupture complicating acute myocardial infarction or as a result of acute ischemic episodes involving the Left circumflex or right coronary Artery, resulting in 'Flash pulmonary edema'. Chronic IMR is primarily a ventricular problem, not a valvular problem, caused by LV remodeling resulting from ischemic cardiomyopathy. Chronic IMR is characterizes by a dynamic nature that may affect the degree of regurgitation and is related to several factor, including LV function and loading conditions. The majority of patients with chronic IMR is asymptomatic and may be incidentally discovered during evaluation for myocardial revascularization. Less commonly, those patients may present with progressive heart failure when MR is moderate to severe. Transthoracic /Transesophageal Echocardiography represents the gold standard for evaluation if IMR. It has been used to establish the diagnosis of IMR as well as to quantify the degree of regurgitation and to identify the underlying mechanism of valve dysfunction to guide any possible therapy. Cardiac MRI has recently emerged as single-pass diagnostic tool that allows evaluation of valvular/ subvalvular and LV geometry, along with myocardial viability, which has recently been shown to be predictive of post-revascularization outcome on IMR. Ischemic Mitral Regurgitation (IMR) continues to be a perplexing clinical problem and controversy continues with regards to optimal therapeutic modality. The authors review in this chapter different diagnostic and therapeutic modalities for chronic IMR with emphasis on the decision making process supported by up to date review of the available evidence.

Chapter 3 - Surgical strategies for the treatment of infective endocarditis (IE) of the mitral valve (MV) remain controversial. MV repair has recently assumed popularity over MV replacement due to its benefits in preserving ventricular function and avoiding the use of a prosthetic valve [1-3] particularly during the active-stage with continued fever, septicemia, septic emboli, or acute heart failure. This chapter outlines current thinking in surgical intervention for MV during active-stage IE.

Chapter 4 - Mitral valve disease is a common disease that requires an accurate evaluation of mitral valve structural changes and their hemodynamic significance. In cases of mitral valve regurgitation, Evaluation of disease severity and its effect on myocardial function plays an important role on choosing the appropriate treatment modality and its timing. When surgical treatment is indicated, pre-operative assessment of MV anatomy is essential for surgical planning and design in patients undergoing MV repair. Although two-dimensional (2D) echocardiography provides precise information regarding MV anatomy, three-dimensional (3D) echocardiography could increase the understanding of MV apparatus and individual scallop identify-cation. Real time 3D (RT3D) transesophageal echocardiogram allows accurate and feasible identification of prolapse or flail of individual segments of MV leaflets during surgery. Echocardiography is also an important tool for management of patients with mitral valve stenosis. To define the best therapeutic strategy in patients with mitral valve stenosis, clinical data and accurate measurements of mitral valve area (MVA) are necessary. Doppler-based methods are heavily influenced by hemodynamic variables, and associated valvular disease. Direct measurements of the MVA could traditionally only be performed using a planimetry traced on 2D echo images. However, this method has multiple limitations; the major one being the correct image plane orientation. RT-3D echocardiography provides a unique 'en-face' view of the complete mitral valve apparatus and has been shown to improve the accuracy of 2D echo MVA planimetry. RT3D echo provides a similari nter-observer variability compared with the pressure half-time method and shows a better inter-observer agreement than 2D echo for the assessment of the pre-valvuloplasty Wilkins score. 2D and 3D echocardiography should be regarded as complementary, not competitive, imaging modalities in patients with complex MV anatomy. Formal 3D echocardiographic training should be encouraged and its use should be expanded use of in routine clinical practice. The authors review in this chapter the clinical uses of 2D and 3D echo-cardiography in assessment of mitral valve disease including up to date literature on this subject.

Chapter 5 - Mitral valve diseases result in structural and functional changes in the mitral complex caused by congenital anomalies or acquired pathogenic factors. The symptoms of mitral valve disease are mitral stenosis or mitral regurgitation. There are a few cases of congenital mitral lesions, and acquired mitral lesions are the most common in underdeveloped countries, particularly in the form of rheumatic mitral valve disease, whereas the most common mitral valve disease in developed countries is mitral valve prolapsed. The earliest diagnostic techniques for mitral lesions were cardio angiography and heart catheterization, but traumatic examinations have gradually been replaced by the ultrasonic cardiogram. Twenty years ago, cardiovascular magnetic resonance (CMR) emerged as the gold standard for assessing heart function. In some developed countries, CMR is also an important supplementary measure for diagnosing and grading mitral lesions. Ultrasonic cardiogram and CMR have their respective advantages and limitations for diagnosing mitral lesions. For example, the ultrasonic cardiogram shows poor repetition, whereas CMR is expensive. In recent years, with the rapid growth of imaging technology, computed tomography (CT) has been used to observe the shape and function of the mitral valve. Currently, CT is not applied widely to clinically diagnose valvular heart disease, and few studies have been conducted except for a few cases of mitral lesions. In this chapter, imaging evaluation of mitral valve disease and related cardiac function changes were reviewed.

Chapter 6 - About 2% of the population in the United States suffers from 'significant' mitral regurgitation (MR). Surgery is indicated for symptomatic patients or asymptomatic patients with decreased left ventricular ejection fraction. Many patients who have MR have considerable comorbidities for high risk surgery, and less invasive approach may be beneficial for these patients. Percutaneous treatment for valvular diseases is attractive because it provides a less traumatic alternative avoiding sternotomy and cardiopulmonary bypass, which means lesser complications and shorter hospital stay. Hence, the concept of percutaneous repair is encouraging and merits attention. An ideal Mitral valve (MV) repair should achieve normal coaptation of the leaflets and maintain leaflet mobility, without injuring the adjacent structures. During the last decade, a considerable progress has been made in the development of transcatheter devices and techniques to treat MR. Some percutaneous techniques for treatment of MR utilize the existing surgical principles, while some are based on novel concepts. These techniques are in various stages of development, ranging from pre-clinical investigation phase to early phase of clinical application. These techniques could be broadly grouped based on the target areas of treatment: annuloplasty (indirect and direct), leaflet repair, and chamber remodeling.

In: Mitral Valve Disease
Editor: Richard R. Heuser
ISBN: 978-1-61942-309-1

Chapter 1

DEGENERATIVE MITRAL VALVE DISEASE

Turki B. Albacker[1], Mazin Alsalihi[2], A. Mark Gillino[3] and Suresh Keshavamurthy[4]

[1]Department of Cardiac Surgery, King Fahad Cardiac Center, King Khalid Medical City, King Saud University Riyadh, Saudi Arabia

[2]Department of Thoracic and Cardiovascular Surgery, Heart and Vascular Institute, Cleveland Clinic Foundation, Cleveland, OH, US

[3]Department of Thoracic and Cardiovascular Surgery, Heart and Vascular Institute, Cleveland Clinic Foundation, Cleveland, IH, US

[4]Clinical AssociateDepartment of Thoracic and Cardiovascular Surgery, Heart and Vascular Institute, Cleveland Clinic Foundation, Cleveland, OH, US

ABSTRACT

Degenerative mitral valve (MV) disease is the most common form of organic non-ischemic MV regurgitation. Myxomatous degeneration commonly involves the annulus, the leaflets and the subvalvular apparatus. Three forms of degenerative mitral valve disease have been described based on the extent and degree of degenerative changes: Barlow's disease, Fibro elastic deficiency and Forme Froste. Quantitative grading of mitral regurgitation is a powerful predictor of the clinical outcome of asymptomatic mitral regurgitation. The combination of symptoms and echocardiographic assessment (severity of regurgitation, left ventricular size and function, left atrial size and pulmonary artery systolic pressure) guides the timing of surgical intervention. MV replacement with either a biologic or mechanical prosthesis used to be the standard of care for surgical treatment of degenerative MV regurgitation. A variety of MV repair techniques have been developed with a success rate of 90% in expert hands at high volume centers. The choice of specific repair technique is based on the segmental analysis of the mitral valve preoperatively using Echocardiography and intra-operatively by direct visualization. The results of surgical treatment of degenerative mitral valve disease are dependent on the extent of the disease, technique used and the preoperative ventricular function. We review in this chapter the pathophysiology of degenerative mitral valve regurgitation, its natural history and echocardiographic assessment of mitral regurgitation caused by degenerative MV disease. This review discusses also different surgical techniques used to treat degenerative MV regurgitation and the results of these techniques supported by up to date review of the literature.

INTRODUCTION

Mitral regurgitation affects more than 2 million people in the USA. Degenerative mitral valve disease represents the most common etiology (60-70%) of mitral valve disease. This disease progresses insidiously, because the heart compensate for increasing regurgitant volume by left atrial enlargement, causes left ventricular overload and dysfunction, and yield poor outcome when it becomes severe. Mitral regurgitation is defined as systolic retrograde flow from the left ventricle into the left atrium. Moderate or severe regurgitation is frequent, its prevalence increases with age, and it was estimated to affect 2.0-2.5 million people in the USA in 2000, which is expected to double by 2030 because of population aging and growth (1). Improved knowledge of clinical outcome of patients with mitral regurgitation resulted in refined surgical indications (2, 3). Hence, mitral regurgitation is a disease in which restoration of life expectancy can often be achieved, an encouraging outcome that emphasizes the importance of early detection, assessment, and prompt consideration for treatment of patients with this condition (2, 3).

The current concepts in the pathophysiology, assessment, and repair of degenerative mitral regurgitation are focusing on the role of valve anatomy in guiding both surgical referral and operative approach; such a strategy will play an important role in the increasing the rate of successful and durable repairs in degenerative mitral valve disease.

Definition of Degenerative Mitral Regurgitation

Degenerative disease is defined as a spectrum of conditions in which infiltrative or dysplastic tissue changes cause elongation or rupture of the mitral valve chorea resulting in leaflet prolapse and associated annular dilatation (4). At one end of the spectrum of degenerative mitral disease is fibro elastic deficiency, characterized by insufficient tissue in a normal sized valve (Figure 1), leaflets are thinned, almost transparent, and chordae are flimsy and thin. Regurgitation is mostly frequently caused by rupture of a single chord associated with a single prolapsing segment, usually P2 resulting in Type II leaflet dysfunction. The prolapsing segment may become distended and thinned by a localized myxomatous process in the chronic setting.

At the opposite end of the spectrum of degenerative mitral regurgitation is Barlow's disease, characterized by marked excess tissue involving multiple leaflet segments in an otherwise large valve (Figure 2). Leaflet tissue is thickened and redundant, with thick, elongated mish-like chordae, which may or may not be ruptured (4).

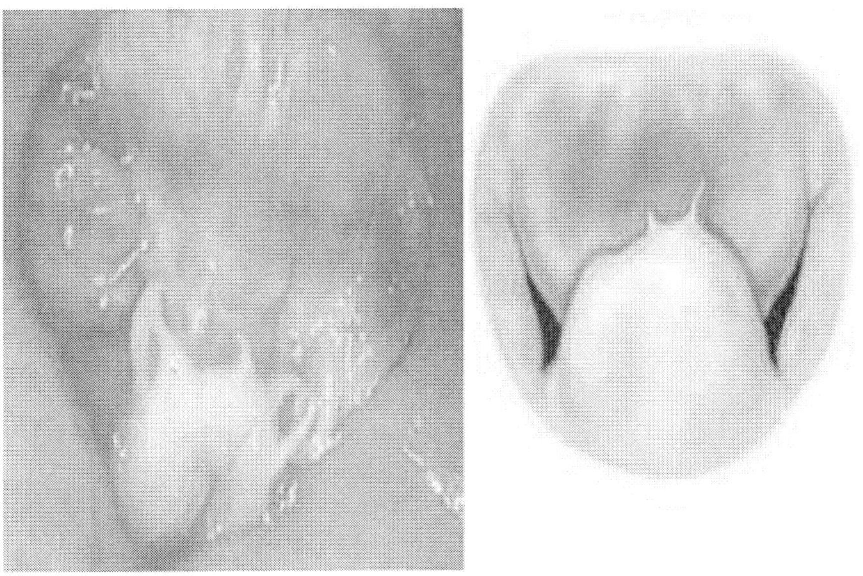

Figure 1. An intra-operative photograph of a valve with fibroelastic deficiency, showing thinned leaflets in a small valve with single segment prolapse, which may or may not be thickened.

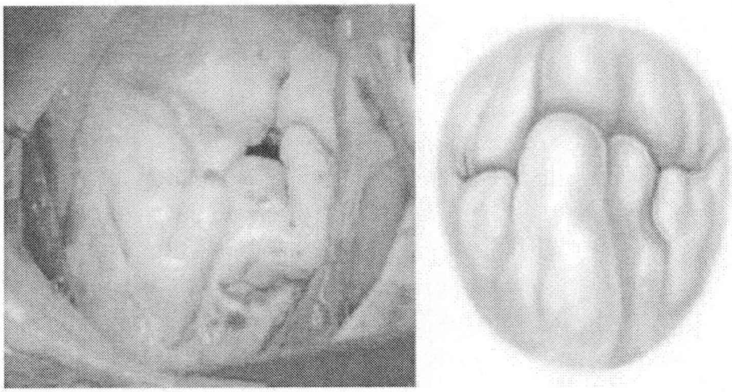

Figure 2. An intra-operative photograph of a typical valve of Barlow's disease, showing thickened leaflets with excess tissue resulting in multi-segment prolapse in a large valve.

Regurgitation is due to multiple areas of prolapse (Type II leaflet dysfunction). Some regurgitant valves occupy a position within the spectrum of fibroelastic deficiency and Barlow's disease, referred to as Forme Fruste of Barlow's disease, as they show areas of excessive and thickened tissue in somewhat smaller valves.

Pathophysiology and Mechanisms

All lesions that cause mitral regurgitation do so by reduction or elimination of the normal coaptation between anterior and posterior mitral leaflets, which normally ensures mitral competences. Consistent anatomical and functional descriptors of mitral lesions are essential to assess surgical reparability but overlapping and poorly defined terminology has caused confusion (Table 1).

Table 1. Etiology and presumed mechanism of degenerative mitral valve regurgitation

Etiology	Presumed mechanism
Annular dilatation	Inadequate leaflet coaptation
Mitral annular calcification (MAC)	Increased rigidity of the annulus leading to impairment of systolic contraction
Myxomatous degeneration	Inadequate coaptation and apposition, with or without flail segment

Degenerative mitral regurgitation is usually related to mitral valve prolapse and rarely to isolated mitral annular calcification. Mitral valve prolapse is an abnormal systolic valve into the left atrium (≥2 mm beyond saddle-shaped annular level) (5). Prolapse might be of moderate magnitude (leaflet tips remain in the left ventricle, i.e. billowing mitral valve) or can be severe (eversion of leaflet tip into left atrium, i.e. flail leaflet-usually caused by ruptured chordae). The main phenotypes of mitral prolapse are diffuse myxomatous degeneration (mitral valve prolapse syndrome or Barlow's disease (6), sometimes with posterior annular translocation into left atrium), or primary flail leaflets with ruptured chordae affecting the posterior leaflet in 70% of cases, and accompanied by myxomatous degeneration localized to the flail segment and generally normal valve morphology elsewhere (7). Myxomatous degeneration remodels valve tissue by increasing the spongiosa layer and valve water content and thickness, with mucopolysaccharide and matrix changes (8), as a functional manifestation of metalloproteinase alterations. These mitral tissue changes and prolapse might be genetically transmitted and X-chromosomal linked (9).

The degree of mitral regurgitation is defined by lesion severity (measured as effective regurgitant orifice [ERO] area) (10) and the yielding volume overload (measured as regurgitant volume [RVol]), but it is also affected by the driving force (left ventricular systolic pressure) and left atrial compliance. Thus, in acute disease, the large regurgitant orifice converts ventricular energy mostly into potential energy (left atrial pressure V-wave) due to non-compliant left-atrium (11). In chronic regurgitation, the enlarged left atrium is compliant, the V-wave is often small, and ventricular energy is converted mostly into kinetic energy (large RVol). This process of atrial enlargement and increased compliance probably explained atrial pressure reduction and clinical improvement after initial heart failure caused by acute mitral regurgitation.

The ERO area is not necessarily fixed and can be dynamic (12). Increased loading or contractility can cause the ERO area to increase or decrease slightly. With valve prolapse, the area is very dynamic, increasing progressively during systole, and is sometimes purely end-diastolic (34). In functional mitral regurgitation, ERO area is dynamic during systole, with large area during short isovolumic contraction and relaxation phases caused by lesser ventricular pressure apposing leaflets (13). The type of regurgitation is also dynamic with decrease loading (14) or inotrope administration, and might disappear with these interventions, whereas exercise most often results in augmentation of ERO area (15). Long-term progression of organic disease is about 5-7 ml per year for RVol and is determined by ERO area progression caused by new lesions or annular dilatation (16). Thus, mitral regurgitation is self-sustained, causing atrial and annular enlargement, which in turn leads to increased ERO area.

The ventricular and atrial consequences of organic mitral regurgitation are initiated by volume overload with increased preload and left ventricular and left atrial enlargement. Impedance to ejection is reduced despite normal or increased vascular resistances, whereas myocardial after load (end-systolic wall stress) is normal with an end-systolic volume that is normal to slightly increased. Thus in degenerative mitral valve, altered left ventricular function might coexist with normal or high ejection fraction (17). Borderline normal ejection fraction, between 50-60%, already implies overt left ventricular dysfunction (18). Ventricular dysfunction should be suspected when end-systolic dimension are large (19), but is often masked by a large ejection volume and is revealed after surgical elimination of mitral regurgitation, with a postoperative average immediate ejection fraction drop of 10% (18). Diastolic ventricular dysfunction is difficult to characterize, but seems to reduce exercise capacity (20).

Table 2. Anatomical lesions and resultant leaflet dysfunction causing mitral regurgitation

Leaflet dysfunction	**Anatomical lesion**
Type I Normal leaflet motion	 Annular dilatation Leaflet perforation
Type II Leaflet prolapse	 Chordal rupture Chordal elongation Papillary muscle rupture
Type III A: Restricted leaflet opening	 Commissural fusion Leaflet thickening Leaflet calcification Chordal fusion
B: Restricted leaflet closure	Chordal thickening Chordal shortening Ventricular dilatation

ANATOMICAL OVERVIEW

Carpentier described a systematic approach for mitral regurgitation, consisting of a "pathophysiological triad". The regurgitant valve is described first by *disease etiology* (e.g. fibroelastic deficiency, Barlow's disease) then by the *primary lesion* (e.g. chordal rupture, annular dilatation); and finally by the resultant *leaflet dysfunction* relating to the motion of leaflet margin (Table 2).

Type II leaflet dysfunction is by far the commonest finding in mitral regurgitation due to degenerative disease. Within the spectrum of degenerative disease, it is important to emphasize that patients may present with different etiologies (e.g. Barlow's or fibroelastic deficiency), multiple different lesions (e.g. chordal elongation or rupture or less commonly restriction, leaflet prolapse, papillary or annular calcification, and annular dilatation), and multiple dysfunctions (Type I, Type II, and Type III), although the primary dysfunction is almost always Type II (excess leaflet motion).

ASSESSMENT

Clinical Features

History and physical examination alone are of limited use in the diagnosis of Mitral Regurgitation, but the severity of symptoms, or evidence of atrial fibrillation, pulmonary hypertension or embolic disease is of direct relevance to the decision of whether and when to refer for surgery. Chronic mitral regurgitation may be asymptomatic for many years.

The most common presenting symptoms are fatigue, decreased exercise tolerance, dyspnea and palpitations. It is important to ask specifically about any previous history of atrial fibrillation, which may not be present at the time of examination. Pulmonary hypertension is suggested by the presence of parasternal heave, and fluid retention is a sign of cor pulmonale.

Clinical features may be helpful in distinguishing between the subtypes of degenerative mitral regurgitation; patients with Barlow's disease are typically younger, with a long history of murmur, compared to those of fibroelastic deficiency who are older, with a relatively short history of mitral insufficiency.

Echocardiograph

Doppler Echocardiography is the main method for assessment of patients with mitral regurgitation. Transthoracic or transesophageal echocardiography provide functional anatomical information that is crucial for assessment of reparability by defining cause, mechanism, presence of calcification, and localization of lesions. Transesophageal echocardiography provides better imaging quality than transthoracic echocardiography but its ability to detect details such as ruptured chordae rarely changes management. Transesophageal echocardiography essentially provides incremental clinically meaningful information (such as reparability) when transthoracic echocardiography is of poor quality or when complex, calcified, or endocarditic lesions are suspected. Thus, transesophageal echocardiography is rarely used on an outpatient basis and is mostly used intra-operatively for lesion verification and to monitor surgical results (21).

Doppler echocardiography provides crucial information about mitral regurgitation severity (Table 3) (22). Comprehensive integration of color-flow imaging and pulsed and continuous wave Doppler echocardiography is necessary because jet-based assessment has major limitations (23). Quantitative assessment of regurgitation is feasible by three methods: *quantitative Doppler* echocardiography based on mitral and aortic stroke volumes (24), *quantitative two-dimensional* echocardiography based on left ventricular volumes, and *flow-convergence analysis* measuring low with color-flow imaging proximal to the regurgitant orifice (proximal isovelociy surface area method; Figure 3) (25). Consistency in all measures of mitral regurgitation severity is essential to appropriately grade disease severity. Hemodynamic assessment is completed with Doppler measurement of cardiac index and pulmonary pressure

Doppler echocardiography also measures left ventricular and left atrial consequences of mitral regurgitation. End-diastolic left ventricular diameter and volume indicate volume overload whereas end-diastolic dimension shows overload and ventricular function. Patients with left ventricular ejection fraction less than 60% or end-systolic diameter of at least 40-45 mm are regarded as having overt left ventricular dysfunction (2). Left atrial diameter indicates volume overload but also conveys important prognostic information. Left atrial volume is recommended as the preferred measure of atrial overload (26), (at least 40 ml/m^2 for severe dilatation) and predicts the occurrence of atrial fibrillation.

Echocardiography is diagnostic, although it must be emphasized that mitral regurgitation is a dynamic condition highly dependent on preload and after load; under conditions of reduced preload or after load, such as under general anesthesia during intra-operative TEE, mitral regurgitation is frequently downgraded, and stress Echo maybe the only means of detecting severe mitral regurgitation in some patients.

Table 3. Gradation of mitral regurgitation by Doppler echocardiography

	Mild	Moderate	Severe
Specific signs	Small central jet <4 cm^2 or <10% of LA, vena contracta width <0·3 cm, no or Minimum flow convergence	MR more than mild, without any criteria for severe MR	Vena contracta width ≥0·7 cm with large central MR jet (area >40% of LA) or with a wall-impinging jet of any size; large flow convergence; systolic reversal in pulmonary veins; prominent Flail leaflet or ruptured papillary muscle
Supportive signs	Systolic dominant flow in pulmonary veins; A-wave dominant mitral inflow; low-density Doppler MR signal; Normal LV size	MR more than mild, but no criteria for Severe MR	Dense, triangular Doppler MR signal; E-wave dominant mitral inflow (>1·2 m/s); enlarged LV and LA, (particularly with Normal LV function)
Quantitative variarle RVol (ml per beat) RF ERO area (cm2)	 <30 <30% <0·20	 30–44; 45–59 30–39%; 40–49% 0·20–0·29; 0·30–0·39	 ≥60 ≥50% ≥0·40

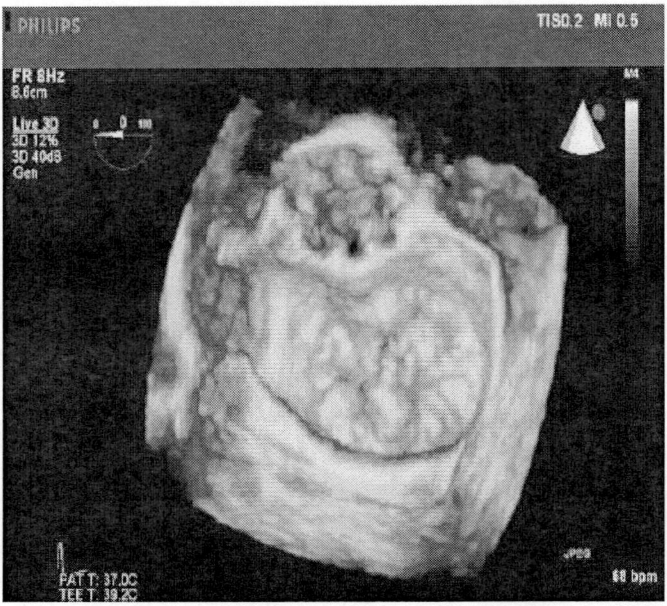

Figure 3. Three-dimensional echocardiography of the mitral valve from the surgeon's view. A flail posterior leaflet is apparent with a ruptured chord.

When mitral regurgitation appears insignificant on pre-bypass intra-operative TEE, it may be helpful to administer vasopressors and volume to recreate physiological conditions same as in awake patient, and then to review the pre-operative trans-thoracic Echo.

Two-dimensional Echo with color Doppler permits accurate determination of the leaflet dysfunction and semi-quantitative assessment of the severity of the mitral regurgitation by maximal jet length and area, the ratio of jet to left atrial area, and vena contracta mapping (Table 3). Regurgitant jet geometry is assessed in multiple views and mitral regurgitation is graded on a scale of 0 to 4+, where 1+ is trace mitral regurgitation and 4+ is severe mitral regurgitation. Color Doppler jet area is affected by jet eccentricity, user and instrumentation factors, and left atrial size (27), potentially leading to variation in estimates of the severity of mitral regurgitation.

Quantitative Doppler grading of mitral regurgitation seeks to standardize assessment of mitral regurgitation. Calculation of regurgitant volume using proximal iso-electric surface area (PISA), vena contracta width and effective regurgitant orifice (ERO), are essential adjuncts in a detailed assessment of mitral regurgitation. An ERO > 40 mm² is acceptable as the cut-off for severe mitral regurgitation in the setting of degenerative disease.

Real-time three dimensional Echo has already yielded insights on the mechanism of the mitral regurgitation and it provides a surgical view of the mitral valve where even subtle areas of prolapse or restriction may be immediately identified (Figure 3) (4).

Exercise Tests

Exercise tests are used to define functional capacity. One in five asymptomatic patients show severe functional limitations during cardiopulmonary exercises (20). Peak oxygen consumption compared with that expected for age, sex, and weight objectively measures functional limitations versus normal reference values. Standard post exercise echocardiography was used to detect exertional ventricular volume increases as a predictor of post-operative left ventricular dysfunction (28), but difficulties in measurement of monoplane ventricular volume hinder this approach. Other stress tests are rarely used.

Computerized Tomographic Angiography (CTA)

This modality is useful to assess patients who are candidates for minimally invasive techniques such as right anterior thoracotomy and robotic mitral valve repair. CTA is important to detect any calcification or tortousity in the ilio-femoral arterial system as well as calcifications in the thoracic and abdominal aorta that may increase the risk of embolization when femoral arterial cannulation is used.

Cardiac Catheterization

This is not consistently used by institutions and might be overused in some. In academic centers, it is rarely used to define hemodynamics, which is usually provided by Doppler echocardiography. Left ventriculography and right heart catheterization are rarely needed for assessment of mitral regurgitation. Conversely, in most patients aged 45 years or older, coronary angiography is routinely done preoperatively.

NATURAL HISTORY

Natural history of degenerative mitral regurgitation has been poorly defined, largely because of limitations in severity assessment. Old studies, before echocardiography, showed a wide range in 5-year survival rates from 27% to 97% probably related to variations in severity (29). Most data were from studies diagnosed with mitral regurgitation due to flail leaflets, most of who had severe regurgitation. Such patients have ventricular enlargement causing the notable volume overload and incur excess overall mortality. Mortality was especially high in patients with class III-IV symptoms but also notable in those with no or minimum symptoms (30). A sudden death rate of 1.8% per year overall varied from as high as 12.0% per year in patients with class III-IV symptoms that had not undergo surgery to 0.8% per year in asymptomatic patients with normal ejection fraction and sinus rhythm (31, 32). Patients in some mitral regurgitation subsets have low mortality, such as young patients (<50years) even with severe mitral regurgitation (33) or those of all ages with initially a moderate disorder (34). Conversely, in a prospective study of asymptomatic patients with long-term follow-up, those with severe regurgitation proven by quantitative measurements showed increased mortality under medical management (34). Thus, older patients ($\geq$ 50 years) with severe (defined as ERO area $\geq$ 40 mm^2) organic mitral regurgitation are at increased risk of death (yearly rates of about 3% for moderate regurgitation *vs.* 6% for the severe organic form). For morbid complications, all studies substantiated the adverse effect of severe regurgitation (33). Patients with flail leaflet (30) and in general those with severe mitral regurgitation (34)had, under medical management, yearly cardiac event rates of 10-12%-including about 9% for heart failure and 5% for atrial fibrillation (35). Within 10 years of diagnosis, cardiac events arise in most patients with severe mitral regurgitation, and death occurs or cardiac surgery is needed in at least 90%, making surgery an almost unavoidable consideration in such patients (36). The risk of stroke is low, but in excess of that expected in old patients and is strongly linked to occurrence of atrial fibrillation, and thus to left-atrial size (36). Predictors of reduced survival under medical management are symptoms (class II-IV), even if transient (30, 31), reduced ejection fraction (31, 33), severe mitral regurgitation with ERO area of 40 mm^2 or more (34). Predictors of cardiac events are atrial fibrillation, left atrial enlargement of at least 40-50 mm diameter (33, 35, 36), flail leafletor large ERO area (34) all markers of severe mitral regurgitation and, during exercise, reduced peak oxygen consumption (20) and possibly reduced right ventricular function (37).

Clinical outcomes after surgery depend on patients-specific, disease-related, and surgery-related factors. Early postoperative mortality is largely affected by age, but improvement of surgical results reduced the risk to about 1% for patients younger than 65 years, 2% for those aged 65-75 years, and 4-5% for older than 75 years (38). Increased surgical risks are also linked to preoperative severe symptoms (39) or heart failure whereas ejection fraction has less effect. Surgery-related determinants of operative risk are governed by mitral reparability, which ensures reduced risk (40); whereas risk is increased with concomitant coronary artery bypass grafting (41). Other associated procedures, such as tricuspid repair or replacement, or those aimed at treatment or prevention of atrial fibrillation need a longer bypass time, which can increase risk. Long-term, patient-related factors continue to affect outcome, particularly coronary disease (41) or reduced renal function. Age determines mortality but restoration of life expectancy is similar in young and old patients (38). After surgery, patients with severe symptoms before surgery continue to have increased mortality despite symptom relief, whereas in those with no or few symptoms, restoration of life expectancy can be achieved (31, 42). Similarly, patients with overt preoperative ventricular dysfunction have increased postoperative mortality, especially with ejection fraction less than 50 % (43). Generally, a 10% early postoperative reduction in ejection fraction happens after elimination of volume overload, whereas end-systolic characteristics (volume, wall stress) are unchanged (43) this reduction is lowest after valve repair (40) and is minimized by preservation of subvalvular apparatus during valve replacement (44). Nevertheless, 25-30% of patients with mitral regurgitation present with postoperative left ventricular dysfunction, especially those with preoperative ejection fraction of less than 60% or end-systolic diameter at least of 40-45 mm (18, 19). Hence, in some centers, prevention of postoperative left ventricular dysfunction relies on performance of early surgery when no sign of left ventricular alteration is present. Coronary disease (even in the absence of angina) increases the risk of left ventricular dysfunction despite the performance of coronary artery bypass grafting (34). Although no clinical trials has compared outcomes of patients randomized to repair versus replacement, observational evidence suggests that the major surgical determinant of improved long-term outcome is valve repair (40), which allows restoration of life expectancy (34) and reduces the risk of heart failure after surgery (45). Although mitral regurgitation can recur after repair, reoperation rates do not differ after repair compared with replacement (40). Thus, mitral valve repair is widely regarded as the preferred mode of correction of organic mitral regurgitation, especially degenerative (40).

The average interval from diagnosis of mitral valve prolapse to the onset of symptoms is approximately 15 years (46), but left ventricular dysfunction frequently occurs before symptoms develop. In patients with severe MR estimates of long-term survival vary widely, but 5-year survival is between 30-95% (46), reflecting the very heterogeneous population included in most series. A review of 348 consecutive patients with chronic MR due to flail leaflet seen at the Mayo Clinic between 1980 and 1989 showed that the incidence of surgery or death at 10 years was 90%, with excess mortality and morbidity in medically treated patients (47). While most deaths related to heart failure, ventricular arrhythmias have been implicated as an important cause of sudden death, particularly (although not exclusively) in symptomatic patients and those with documented left ventricular dysfunction (31).

Management

The natural history of degenerative mitral regurgitation emphasizes the importance of treatment of patients with severe regurgitation. Because the effects of various treatments on survival have not been tested in randomized clinical trials, the value of any approach is estimated on the basis of outcome studies (2).

Medical Treatment

Aims to prevent the progression of degenerative disease. Prevention of endocarditis is directed at forestalling catastrophic infectious complications and sudden mitral regurgitation progression associated with endocarditis (2).

Diuretics often reduce or eliminate symptoms of disease but such improvement should not unduly reassure physicians. Patients who had transiently severe symptoms and improved with treatment continue to be at higher risk and should be promptly assessed for surgery (30).

Treatment of degenerative mitral regurgitation with vasodilators has been advocated on the basis of experimental studies showing reductions in acute RVol and even ERO area with blood pressure reduction (90). Acutely ill patients with mitral regurgitation, benefit from vasodilator treatment. However, despite some encouraging data (48), translation to chronic treatment of organic disease is unresolved because reported series were small, rarely randomized, and contradictory in conclusions (49).

Activation of the tissue (not systemic) renin-angiotensin system was shown in organic mitral regurgitation. Consistent pilot studies suggest potential benefits of drugs blocking tissue renin-angiotensin system to stabilize organic mitral regurgitation severity and consequences (50-51). The effect of such treatments on clinical outcome remains to be shown. B-blockade in degenerative mitral regurgitation has only been tested in animal models and remains conjectural (52).

Indications for Surgery

Factors determining timing of surgery for isolated MR in the current American college of Cardiology and American Heart Association (ACC/AHA) guidelines include symptoms, left ventricular ejection fraction, left ventricular end systolic dimension, atrial fibrillation, and pulmonary hypertension (53). While there is a consensus that patients in whom mitral repair is feasible should undergo surgery before evidence of left ventricular decompensation, the poorer outcomes associated with mitral replacement mean that asymptomatic patients with severe mitral regurgitation but preserved left ventricular function should not undergo surgery if replacement rather than repair is the likely operative outcome (53).

Symptoms

The annual mortality of medically treated patients on the New York Heart Association (NYHA) functional class III or IV, even if the patients only transiently deteriorated into one of these classes, was shown in one study to be as high as 34% (47). NYHA functional class is also an independent predictor of postoperative mortality and left ventricular dysfunction (39). Severe symptoms of congestive heart failure, whether transient or persistent, indicate the need for surgical intervention, and a cogent case has been made for operating earlier in less symptomatic patients (39). Stress testing may be required to demonstrate true NYHA status in a limited subset of apparently asymptomatic patients (2). Current ACC/AHA guidelines recommend that asymptomatic and NYHA class I and II patients with severe mitral regurgitation should be referred for surgery based on deterioration in left ventricular function (class I), atrial fibrillation or raised pulmonary artery pressures (class IIa).

Left Ventricular Ejection Fraction

The strongest predictor of outcome after surgery for chronic mitral regurgitation is the pre-operative left ventricular ejection fraction (39, 43). Despite the fact that the presence of mitral regurgitation means left ventricular ejection fraction underestimates the degree of left ventricular dysfunction, pre-operative ejection fraction has been shown to be a significant predictor of post-operative ventricular function (39, 43), functional status and long-term survival (Figure 4) (54). ACC/AHA guidelines recommend surgery for patients with severe mitral regurgitation and a left ventricular ejection fraction < 60%, irrespective of symptoms, and suggest that patients with ejection fraction > 60 % should be monitored with serial echocardiograms. Surgery should be undertaken if there is evidence of progressive deterioration in left ventricular ejection fraction (2).

Left Ventricular End Systolic Diameter

Left ventricular end systolic diameter and left ventricular end systolic volume index are simple, reproducible measures of left ventricular function that can be obtained non-invasively, and have the advantage that they are relatively independent of hemodynamic status. Pre- operative Left Ventricular End Systolic Diameter (LVESD) is an independent predictor of post-operative ventricular function: a Left Ventricular End Systolic Diameter of 45 mm represents the value above which patients are highly likely to have abnormal post-operative left ventricular function (18).

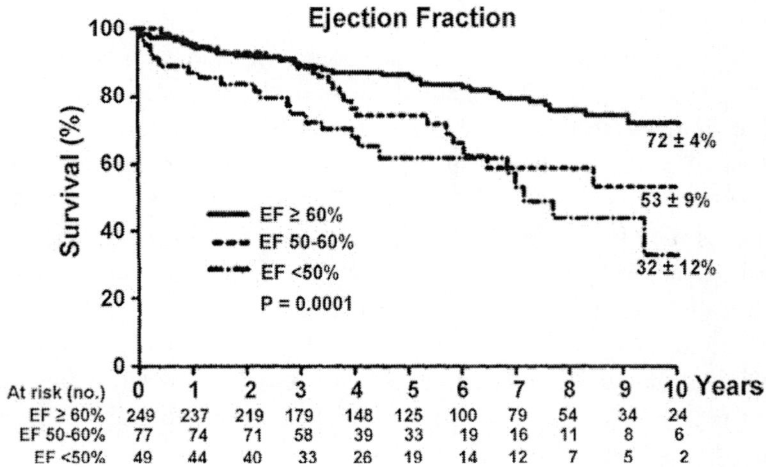

Figure 4. Pre-operative ejection fraction has been shown to be a significant predictor of long-term survival after mitral repair. Figure from Ref. [40].

Pre-operative left ventricular end systolic volume index has been shown to be inversely correlated with post-operative left ventricular function and survival, with a left ventricular end systolic volume index >50 ml/m^2 predictive of persistent of post-operative left ventricular dilatation (43). ACC/AHA guidelines recommend surgery for patients with severe mitral regurgitation and left ventricular end systolic diameter > 40 mm, irrespective of symptom status (class I) (2).

Atrial Fibrillation

Atrial fibrillation, which occurs in almost a third of medically treated patients with mitral regurgitation (47), carries significant morbidity and mortality. Chronic atrial fibrillation occurs almost exclusively in patients with a left atrial diameter > 40 mm, and less likely than recent onset or intermittent fibrillation to be successfully converted to sinus rhythm by surgery (55). For this reason ACC/AHA guidelines recommend consideration of surgery in patients with severe mitral regurgitation and atrial fibrillation irrespective of left ventricular function and symptomatic status (class IIa). Surgical ablation is now a standard adjunct to mitral repair as it increases the number of patients that are in sinus rhythm post-operatively, as well as freedom from anti-coagulation and its associated morbidity and mortality (56).

Elevated Pulmonary Artery Pressures

Pulmonary artery hypertension is associated with significant increase in post-operative early mortality, poorer functional status and reduced long-term survival (57). A marker of severe left ventricular diastolic dysfunction and of the severity of mitral regurgitation, it is associated with poorer post-operative indices of left ventricular function (43). ACC/AHA guidelines recommend consideration of surgery in patients with severe mitral regurgitation and pulmonary artery pressures > 50 mmHg at rest or > 60 mmHg during exercise irrespective of left ventricular function and symptomatic status (class IIa).

Timing of Surgery

The contrast between the substantial morbidity and mortality associated with chronic severe mitral regurgitation and the excellent outcomes associated with mitral valve repair in degenerative disease has led experienced groups to adopt a policy of early intervention in patients with degenerative disease, before onset of symptoms, atrial fibrillation, left ventricular dysfunction or pulmonary hypertension. This approach is supported by retrospective observational study of over 400 patients with severe degenerative mitral regurgitation which identified an effective regurgitant orifice area of > 40 mm^2 as the single most important predictor of adverse outcome during follow-up (34). The results largely of this study lead ACC/AHA Guidelines to recommend strong consideration of surgery in asymptomatic patients with normal ventricular function and severe chronic mitral regurgitation as long as mitral valve repair was highly likely (class IIa).

On the contrary of that, Rosenhek et al found that over half of patients with severe mitral regurgitation survived for eight years before developing acceptable indications for surgery, with overall survival not significantly different to expected survival with this approach (33). This led the European Guideline Committee to down grade the indication for surgery in these patients to class IIb. There are several potential reasons for the differences between those two series. The primary reason is probably the difference in etiology in the patient's cohorts. Enriquez-Sarano's group had a mean age of 63 years, with less than 10% of those undergoing surgery receiving a valve replacement, which is typical of fibroelastic deficiency. In contrast Rosenhek's patients had a mean age of 58 years, and 17% of those undergoing surgery received a valve replacement, which is more suggestive of Barlow's disease. Patients with Barlow's disease are more likely to experience a long period of event free survival before developing symptoms, atrial fibrillation, ventricular dysfunction or pulmonary hypertension, and watchful waiting is therefore perhaps a more appropriate strategy in this group. In contrast patients with fibroelastic deficiency are more likely to experience adverse events early during follow-up (and more likely to undergo successful valve repair) and a strategy of early mitral valve repair is certainly reasonable.

Surgical Options

Mitral valve repair offers superior long-term survival, freedom from cardiac morbidity, and quality of life in patients with severe mitral regurgitation compared to medical management and mitral valve replacement (34, 58), which makes it the treatment of choice in these patients (53). Mitral valve repair is the only treatment that restores normal life expectancy to otherwise healthy patients with advanced degenerative mitral valve disease (34). Although some studies report repair rate of 90% (59), repair rates in developed countries continue to average around 50% (1, 60). Surgical options for mitral valve repair include full sternotomy, upper partial sternotomy, right anterior thoracotomy or Robotic mitral valve repair.

Repair Techniques

Successful mitral valve repair includes four critical components: (1) accurate assessment of the mechanism of valvular dysfunction; (2) consistent and excellent exposure of the mitral valve; (3) precise application of repair techniques; and (4) intra-operative assessment of the results of repair.

Valve Analysis

A surgical valve analysis is the first step of the operation. Usually the anterior scallop of the posterior leaflet (P1) is free from prolapse and is used as a reference point to compare all other segments. With the help of nerve hooks passed around chordae, the free edge of A1 is compared to A2, then A3, P1, P2 and P3. The findings of the systematic valve analysis should be correlated with those of the intra-operative echocardiography. The specific repair technique applied depends primarily upon the site of prolapse. All leaflet and chordal repair techniques are accompanied by incorporation of an annuloplasty. In patients with degenerative disease, durability does not appear to be strongly influenced by type of prosthetic annuloplasty. Therefore, in such patients, we generally favor a posterior flexible band placed from trigone to trigone.

Posterior Prolapse

Approximately 75% of patients with mitral regurgitation caused by degenerative disease have isolated prolapse of the posterior leaflet, most commonly the P2 segment (middle scallop). The classic technique for managing this is quadrangular resection, with or without sliding repair 61). The sliding repair was developed to reduce the risk of post-repair SAM in the setting of excessive leaflet tissue and/or a small, hyperdynamic left ventricle 62).

Quadrangular Resection

The prolapsed area of the posterior leaflet is identified. 2-0 stay sutures are passed around normal chordae on each side of the prolapsed area. These stay sutures limit the prolapsed area and they improve the exposure. A gentle traction on the stay sutures will expose the prolapsed area well. The quadrangular resection is performed. It is advisable to leave 0.5 cm of tissue on both sides of the resection to reduce the extent of resection. This will leave, at the end of the operation, a 1 cm of free edge on the posterior leaflet unsupported by chordae, which is compatible with good function of the posterior leaflet. It is necessary to pay attention to the base of the resection; the annulus must be cleaned from any mucoid or calcific deposit to facilitate the next steps of the operation. In case of normal posterior leaflet height, a 2-0 suture is placed through the mitral annulus 0.5 cm away from the base of the quadrangular resection on both sides. Tying this suture plicates the annulus (Figure 5), it is important that as a result, the two leaflet remnants come in close apposition with a little overlap (63).

When there is excess tissue and the posterior leaflet height is greater than 2 cm, a sliding leaflet plasty is necessary to reduce the height of the posterior leaflet to minimize the risk of SAM (Figure 6A). The posterior leaflet is detached from the annulus at a distance, which is approximately twice as much as the width of the resected area. When the excess of tissue is large, both sides of the posterior leaflet may be detached from the annulus. When the excess of tissue is more localized, only one side may have to be detached. In any case, the length of the detachment should be at least twice as much as the width of the resection. 2-0 annulus sutures are easily placed at the level of the detached posterior leaflet, since the mitral annulus is well exposed.

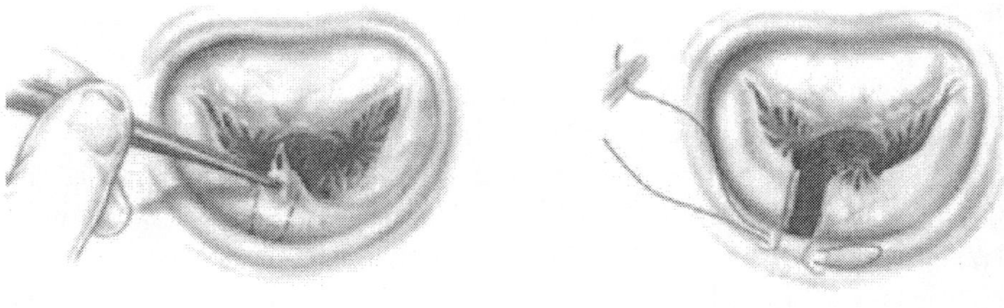

Figure 5.

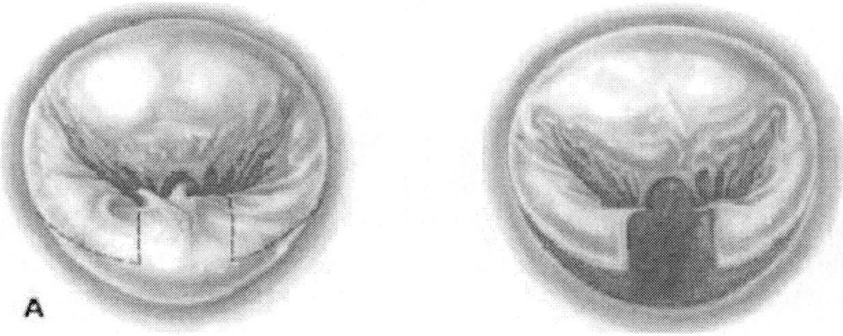

Figure 6A.

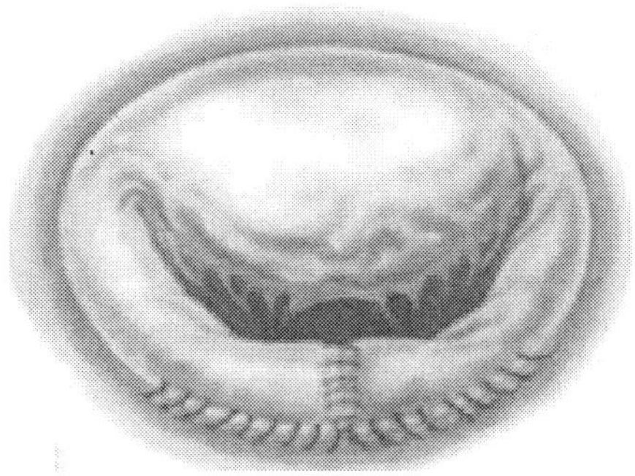

Figure 6B.

The posterior leaflet remnants are reattached to the annulus with a running 4-0 monofilament. Care has to be taken to start the sliding plasty from the beginning of the suture to ensure that tension on the posterior leaflet is regularly distributed and that the gap of the posterior leaflet is adequately covered. It is important that the posterior leaflet remnants come in close apposition with a little overlap. The two leaflet remnants are affixed to each other with a running 5-0 monofilament (Figure 6B). It is important that this suture is performed without any tension (63).

Triangular Resection

In the patient with segmental posterior leaflet prolapse, mitral regurgitation is caused by lack of coaptation at the site of chordal rupture or elongation. Therefore, it is logical to target the prolapsing free edge of the leaflet when addressing this problem. A triangular resection entails resection of the portion of the free edge that prolapses, with incisions in the leaflet angled toward one another as the incision approaches the annular level (Figure 7A) (64). No annular plication sutures are necessary as in a standard quad-rangular resection; this simplifies the procedure and reduces the risk of circumflex artery distortion or kinking (Figure 7B). After triangular resection, care should be exercised not to use too small an annuloplasty, as this may increase the risk of SAM (65). We most frequently employ a posterior flexible band of labeled size 34 to 38 mm. In our clinical practice, we have generally replaced standard quadrangular resection and sliding repair with triangular resection and folding plasty, respectively; these 2 simplified techniques for correction of posterior leaflet prolapse reduce the number of surgical maneuvers and thereby decrease operative time.

Folding Plasty

The folding plasty is used to treat posterior leaflet prolapse when there is a high risk of SAM, replacing the sliding repair in most of these cases (66). The prolapsing portion of the posterior leaflet is resected as for a quadrangular resection, leaving tall posterior leaflet remnants on either side. A suture is passed through the mid-portion of the cut leaflet edge on each side, and this suture is then passed through the annulus at the mid-portion of the area of resection; this maneuver reduces the posterior leaflet height (Figure 8A). If necessary, suture placement is modified to ensure that the leaflet remnants are of similar height. Leaflet tissue is then approximated to the annulus, closing the gap at the annular level and uniformly reducing the height of the posterior leaflet in this region. The leaflet edges are re-approximated in the middle (Figure 8B) and an annuloplasty completes the repair.

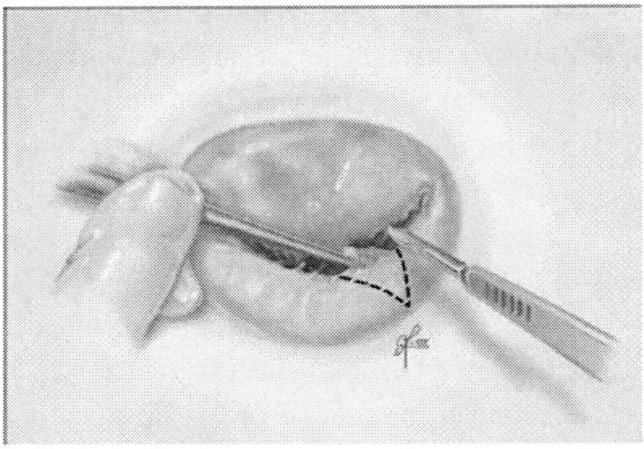

Figure 7A.

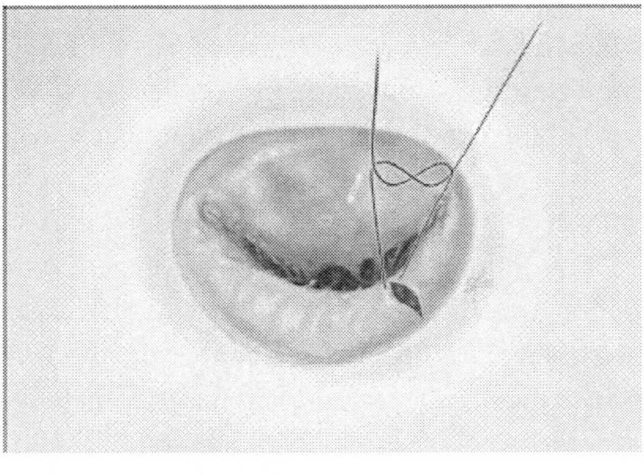

Figure 7B.

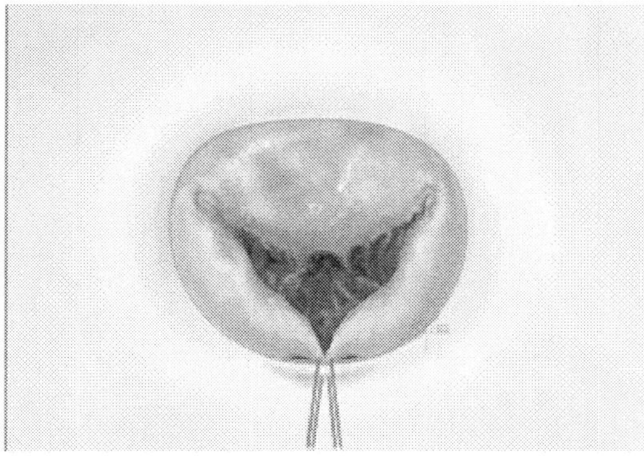

Figure 8A.

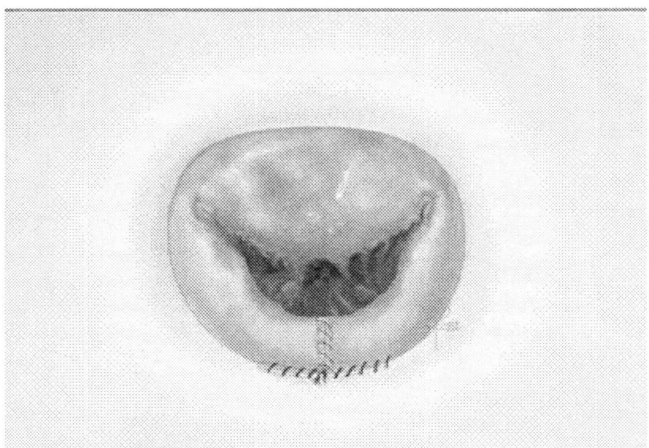

Figure 8B.

Anterior Prolapse

Correction of anterior leaflet prolapse is traditionally more challenging than is correction of posterior leaflet prolapse. Classic techniques for management of anterior leaflet prolapse include chordal transfer, which usually requires manipulation of the posterior leaflet, chordal shortening, which is associated with reduced durability, and triangular resection. Management of anterior prolapse by creation of artificial chordae or the edge-to-edge repair simplifies the procedure.

Artificial Chordae

Artificial chordae are usually constructed of ePTFE (Gore-Tex, W.L. Gore and Assoc, Flagstaff, AZ). The key challenge with creation of artificial chordae is determination of chordal length, and there are many techniques for estimating chordal length (67, 68).

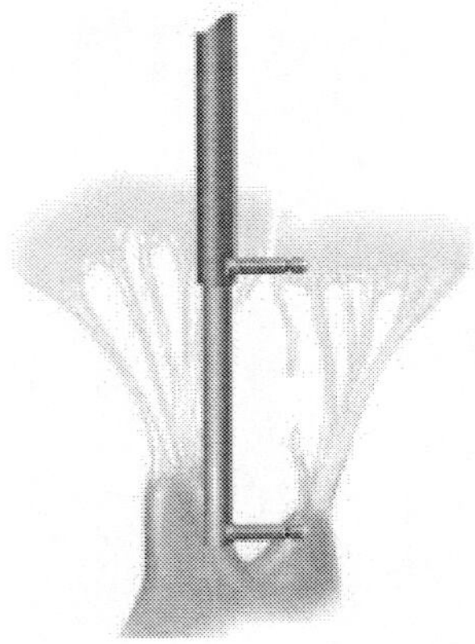

Figure 9A.

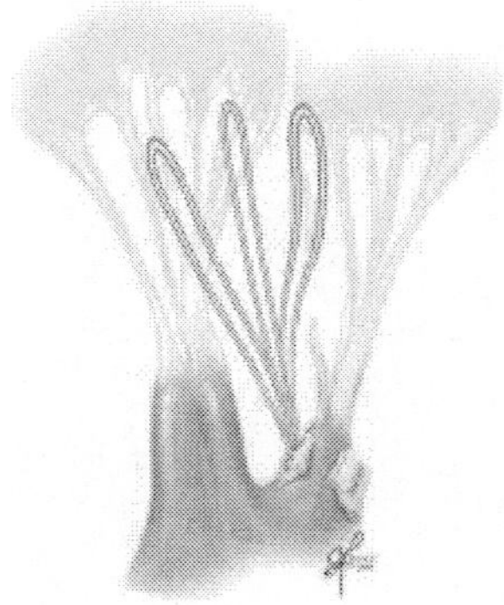

Figure 9B.

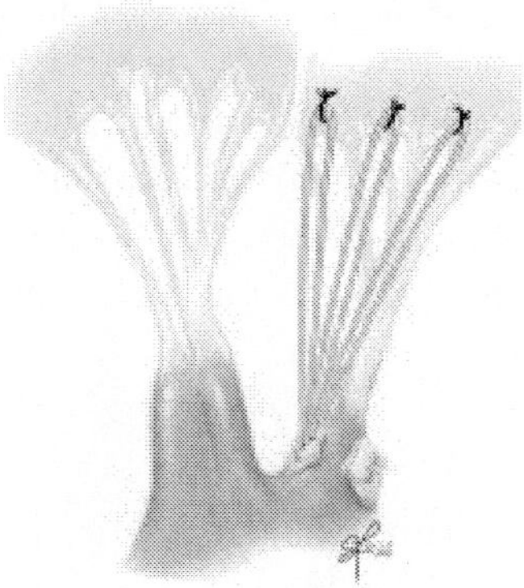

Figure 9C.

We favor use of a caliper for direct measurement and construction of chordal loops, as described by Von Uppell and Mohr (67). With this technique, the caliper is used to measure the length of a normal chord or, if there is no reference chord, the distance from the papillary muscle head to the annulus (Figure 9A). Chordal loops of this length are constructed and affixed to a papillary muscle (Figure 9B); for repair of anterior prolapse, length is most commonly 22 to 24 mm. Finally, the loops are affixed to the free edge of the prolapsing leaflet with a Gore-Tex suture (Figure 9C). This technique may also be applied for correction of posterior leaflet prolapse.

Chordal Transfer

In this technique, the secondary chordae are transferred to the primary position to replace the ruptured or elongated primary chordae (69). Good results have been achieved with this technique but it is unclear why the secondary chordae would be spared from the disease and strong enough to support the repair.

Chordal Transposition

A quadrangular segment of the posterior leaflet attached to both its primary as well secondary chordae is separated from the posterior leaflet and reattached to the edge of the prolapsed segment of the anterior leaflet. The defect in the posterior leaflet is closed primarily or with a sliding plasty. This technique is usually used when there is an isolated prolapsed segment of the anterior leaflet and adequate tissues on the posterior leaflet with normal looking chordae.

Chordal Shortening

This technique has been abandoned due to the high recurrence rate of MR. This failure is related to the use of the same elongated chordae, which are principally weak to start with leading to rupture or further elongation when exposed to stress.

Edge-to-Edge Repair

Described by Alfieri and coworkers, the edge-to-edge repair is the simplest maneuver for correction of prolapse (70). With this technique, the prolapsing segment of the anterior leaflet is sutured to normal posterior leaflet directly opposite, ensuring coaptation and preventing prolapse. Sutures are taken several millimeters deep into the leaflet and span the entire region of prolapse. The stitch should normally not exceed 1 cm in length.

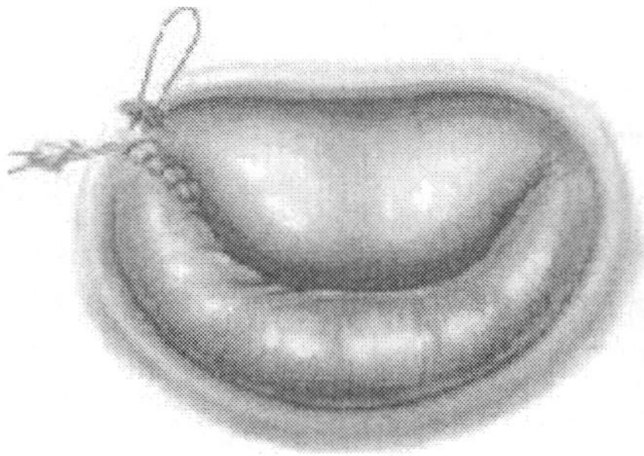

Figure 10.

Of note, the edge-to-edge technique can also be employed to manage posterior prolapse and bileaflet prolapse; however, it is rarely our primary repair technique. An important point of the surgical technique is ourstrong belief that the stitch should be placed only with myxomatousvalves, so as to avoid producing mitral stenosis, as has beenthe case with ischemic MR (71). This technique is a very valuable adjunct in patientswho have the potential for systolic anterior motion of the mitralvalve (72).

Commissural Prolapse

Commissuroplasty is a simple and reproducible solution for management of commissural prolapse involving the anterior leaflet, posterior leaflet, or both leaflets (73). The edge of the prolapsing segment is sutured to the free edge of the opposite leaflet (Figure 10). A relatively large annuloplasty device is employed to avoid mitral stenosis.

Bileaflet Prolapse

Bileaflet prolapse is often a consequence of Barlow's disease. Management of this entity depends upon valve pathology. Nearly all of these patients have excessive leaflet tissue and annular dilatation. In many patients with bileaflet prolapse, leaflet prolapse is asymmetric, and the predominant lesion is prolapse of the middle scallop of the posterior leaflet, producing an anteriorly directed jet of mitral regurgitation. In such cases, mitral valve repair is most often achieved by triangular resection of the middle scallop and insertion of an annuloplasty device. In selected patients with symmetric bileaflet prolapse, a central jet of mitral regurgitation, and no flail, repair can frequently be accomplished by insertion of a large annuloplasty device (typically labeled size 36 or greater); this reduces annular diameter and increases leaflet coaptation. However, in patients with severe bileaflet prolapse it is often necessary to address both leaflets, necessitating a combination of repair techniques (i.e. resection and sliding repair for the posterior leaflet, artificial chordae for the anterior leaflet, and annuloplasty to increase leaflet coaptation).

Remodeling Ring Annuloplasty

Remodeling the annulus by ring annuloplasty after mitral valve repairis essential to a complete and long-lasting repair (74). Different types of rings have been used for repair of degenerative mitral valves. There is some evidence to suggest thatflexible rings and C-shaped rings are associated with decreased incidence of postoperative SAM (75). However, these findings are not supported by prospective randomized studies. The critical technical aspects of ring annuloplasty are the relative upsizing ofthe ring and a secure attachment to the trigone area of theanterior mitral leaflet. The height of the anterior leaflet from the annulus to the highest point on the leaflet when it is stretchedis the most important criterion for sizing, a concept originally espoused by Carpentier (76). This height of the leaflet is the critical dimension that must be carefully measured so that duringsystole there is minimal redundancy that may lead to SAM. Usinginter-trigonal sizing may, in fact, downsize the ring and cause eithersystolic anterior motion or ring dehiscence because of the huge disparity between ring size and annulus size. Other technical aspects of ring implantation that are important include avoiding circumflex artery compromise, atrioventricular dissociation, or dehiscence of the ring. Implantation of currently available annuloplasty rings requires the placement of mattress sutures, parallel to the annulus, at the conjunction of the posterior leaflet and the annulus. Radially oriented bites are to be avoidedbecause by definition they exert radial stresses and thus willpull to some extent on the circumflex artery. Bites should bedeep with the needle entering the annulus, then into the left ventricular cavity, and then coming out on the atrial side again. Of paramount importance is the requirement that the plane ofthe needle bite should be orthogonal to the annular plane.

Mitral Valve Replacement

The indications for mitral valve replacement are variable andundergoing evolution. Common conditions encountered are Mitral stenosis, complex mitral regurgitation, combined stenosis and regurgitation. However with increasing use of reparative techniques, particularly for mitral regurgitation, replacementor repair of a mitral valve often depends on the experienceof the operating surgeon. Current indications for valve replacement pertain to those types of valve problems that are unlikely tobe repaired by most surgeons or which have been shown to havepoor long-term success after reconstruction. Choice of valves are either mechanical or bioprosthetic valves. Of the mechanical valves bileaflet valves, tilting disc valves and ball and cage valves are available; the important factor to be weighed when using mechanical valves is to consider if the patient is a candidate for life long anticoagulation with Coumadin. Bioprosthetic valves are either porcine or pericardial valves. They form the mainstay for replacement. The advantage is that there is no need for mandatory anticoagulation for the valve itself. The disadvantage in the long term is the potential need for re-operation for structural valve degeneration. Homograft mitral valves have been used but the results have not been very encouraging.

RESULTS

Mitral Valve Repair vs. Replacement

Mitral valve repair is associated with low rates of operativemortality (1 to 3%). Data are lacking fromrandomized trials comparing replacement with repair. In a recent meta-analysis of 29 observationalstudies, the early (30-day) rates of operativemortality and longer-term mortality weresignificantly lower after repair than after replacement; however, the analyses were not adjustedfor age or coexisting conditions (77). The apparent survival benefits of mitral-valve repair, versus replacement, are limited to patients with posterior-leaflet disease (77). The outcome after repair is best when intraoperative trans-esophageal echocardiography shows no more thanmild mitral regurgitation at the conclusion of surgery. The decision to proceed with repair rather than replacement is also influenced by other clinical considerations, including the reduced likelihood of a need for long-term anticoagulation therapy after repair as compared with replacement. However, anticoagulation therapy may be required after repair if atrial fibrillation persists or develops or if the patient has a thromboembolic event. After mitral-valve repair, the 15-year incidence of thromboembolic complications exceeds 20% (78). In an observational study comparing various surgeries, the 10-year rate of stroke was 10% with mitral-valve repair, 12% with bioprosthetic valve replacement, and 23% with mechanical-valve replacement; the rate was higher than expected only for the mechanical valve replacement. The risk of thromboembolic events was lower among patients with mitral valve repair than among those with mechanical valves after the first 6 months after surgery (79). At the Cleveland Clinic Foundation, from 1985 to 1997, 1,072 patients with degenerative mitral valve diseasehad isolated primary valve repair for mitral insufficiency. There were three hospital deaths (0.3%). Ten-year actuarial survivalwas 81%. Risk factors for late death included anteriorleaflet prolapse, chordal shortening, annuloplasty alone, older age, renal dysfunction, and atrial fibrillation. At 10 years, freedom from thromboembolism was 88%, from endocarditis 99%, from anticoagulant-related hemorrhage 99%, and from reoperation 93%. Of the 30 patients who required reoperation for late mitral valvedysfunction, 16 (53%) had repair failure secondary toprogressive degenerative disease. Anterior leaflet prolapse, chordal shortening, annuloplasty alone, leafletresection without annuloplasty, and no Intraoperativeechocardiogram increased the risk of late reoperation. The risk of endocarditis is lower among patients who undergo repair (approximately 1.5% at 15 years) (78) than among those who undergo replacement (0.3% to 1.2% per year, with similar rates for mechanical and bioprosthetic valves) (79). The rate of recurrent mitral regurgitation that is more than moderate in severity is 2 to 4% per year in large series at high-volume surgical centers (78). The rate of reoperation, performed in most cases for recurrent mitral regurgitation, is 0.5 to 1.5% per year (78, 80).

Posterior Leaflet Prolapse vs. Anterior Leaflet or Bileaflet Prolapse

The results of repair are also highly dependent on the anatomy of the valve and the experience of the surgeon. Repair of the anterior leaflet is more difficult technically, because chordal transfer or placement of artificial chords is often required. Reoperation rates are higher after repair of an anterior leaflet than after repair of a posterior leaflet, and the rate of long-term survival is lower. The overall rates of reoperation are similar with repair and with replacement of the mitral valve (77).

Chordal Shortening vs. Chordal Transfer or Neochordal Implantation for Anterior Leaflet Prolapse

Elongated chordae are by definition structurally weakenedwith loss of the central collagen core and are likely predisposedto elongation or rupture. It is unknown to what degree stresson the chordae is changed after shortening and what effect residualMR has on the generated stress. The operation is technically more difficult, and it may be that the combination of an imperfectly shortened, inherently weak chordae is at increased risk for rupture. The relatively early and rapid progression to severe MR in the failed repair group would support this contention.

Chordal transfer is reproducible and durable method of repairing anterior leaflet prolapse with 96% 5-year freedom from reoperation. The reason chordal transfer is more durable than chordal shorteningis unknown. Posterior chordal transfer usually includes multipleprimary and secondary chordae and may, therefore, have a mechanical advantage to reduce and evenly distribute the generated stress. Supporting this theory is a recent finite element analysis ofstress on chordae adjacent to a ruptured chordae. Only afterfour artificial chordae were used for reconstruction was stresson the non-ruptured chordae reduced to normal levels (81). With neochordal implantation, the repair is not based on myxomatous chords, which can predispose to late chordal rupture, and because chordal support is actually augmented by the Gore-Tex material, the late failure/reoperation rate has been exceedingly low (2 to 3% over 10 years of follow-up). The subsequent endocarditis rate has been around 1% (a real advantage of repair over replacement), and moderate mitral regurgitation recurrence treated medically has occurred in less than 2%. Together with an operative mortality approaching zero, neochordal implantation currently is the preferred method in treating anterior leaflet or bileaflet prolapse. There are multiple techniques for measuring the optimum length of the neochordae and they are usually based on the adjacent normal chords. Some surgeons advocate pre-formed multiple loops to achieve good coaptation.

MINIMALLY INVASIVE APPROACHES FOR DEGENERATIVE MITRAL VALVE SURGERY

Partial upper Sternotomy

Partial upper sternotomy is performed through a small midline incision (8-10 cm) and Ted to the left 4th intercostal space. Arterial cannulation is performed directly in the ascending aorta and venous drainage is done directly via the aorta and SVC/IVC. Unlike with traditional full sternotomy the approach to the mitral valve is via the trans-septal route and can also use the dome of the left atrium for good exposure.

Anterior Mini-Thoracotomy

This approach is done through 6-8 cm sub-mammary incision at the 4th intercostal space anteriorly. CPB is installed using femoral artery and femoral vein cannulation with the use of vacuum assisted venous drainage. The approach to the mitral valve is through a left atriotomy.

Robotic MV Surgery

Robotic surgery is done using the da Vinci surgical system. The surgeon sits at the console and the robot is positioned at the operating table. Robotically assisted MV repair represents the least invasive form of MV surgery without a compromise in quality ofvalve repair or patient safety, and should therefore be considered for all patients with severe myxomatous MV disease and posterior leaflet prolapse. Ongoing refinements of robotic instrumentation and development of ancillary technologies will facilitate wider adoption of this technique in contemporary surgical practice (82).

Percutaneous Approaches

Valvular edge-to-edge attachment mimics the surgical procedure proposed by Alfieri and colleagues (83), creating a tissue bridge between anterior and posterior leaflets. Percutaneously, this procedure uses a clip or sutures deployed through trans-septal catheterization. Experimental studies have shown success and reliable clip or suture placement through the transseptal approach. Early trials also suggest safety and feasibility with close echo - cardiographic guidance in centers with much experience of interventional valvular procedures. Data for how well this intervention works are preliminary but encouraging (84), suggesting that more than 80% of patients can be discharged from hospital with a clip and mild or little regurgitation. The edge-to-edge technique has important limitations. First, the application of this technique is restricted to localized prolapse of the central segment of the anterior and posterior leaflets. Second, annular dilatation is not addressed by the procedure and might cause residual regurgitation.

Annuloplasty aimed at reduction of annular dilatation is under investigation, mostly with coronary sinus cinching. Technically, stabilization of material with sufficient constraining force to obtain more than 20%

diameter reduction is a challenge. Most devices are composed of anchoring devices placed in the distal and proximal coronary sinus and an intermediate tensioning or supporting element. Experimentally, reduction of mitral regurgitation is achievable (85), but clinical results are preliminary (86). Feasibility through a jugular approach and safety seem to be acceptable. Potential limitations are those of annuloplasty (incomplete valve tenting correction) and those of coronary sinus approach that might reduce only part of the annular circumference with effectiveness limited by the 1-2 cm sinus-annular distance. Because of safety concerns related to proximity of the coronary sinus and circumflex artery with potential artery compression, Non-coronary sinus approaches to annuloplasty and percutaneous ventricular remodeling-constraint devices are being investigated. On the basis of the success of balloon valvuloplasty for mitral stenosis, percutaneous treatment of mitral regurgitation is expected to be successful but this success will necessitate complex development that needs strong cardiologist-engineer collaboration and rigorous assessment.

References

[1] Lung B, Baron G, Butchart EG, et al. A prospective survey of patients with valvular heart disease in Europe: the Euro heart survey on valvular heart disease. *Euro Heart* J 2003; 24: 1231–43.

[2] Bonow RO, Carabello BA, Kanu C, et al. ACC/AHA 2006 guidelines for the management of patients with valvular heart disease: a report of the American College of Cardiology/American Heart Association Task Force on Practice Guidelines (writing committee to revise the 1998 Guidelines for the Management of Patients With Valvular Heart Disease): developed in collaboration with the Society of Cardiovascular Anesthesiologists: endorsed by the Society for Cardiovascular Angiography and Interventions and the Society of Thoracic Surgeons. *Circulation* 2006; 114: e84–231.

[3] Vahanian A, Baumgartner H, Bax J, et al. Guidelines on the management of valvular heart disease: the Task Force on the Management of Valvular Heart Disease of the European Society of Cardiology. *Euro Heart J* 2007; 28: 230–68.

[4] Anyanwu AC, Adams DH. Etiologic classification of degenerative mitral valve disease: Barlow's disease and fibroelastic deficiency. *Semin Thorac Cardiovasc Surg* 2007;19 (2):90–6.

[5] Levine R, Triulzi M, Harrigan P, Weyman A. The relationship of mitral annular shape to the diagnosis of mitral valve prolapses. *Circulation* 1987; 75: 756–67.

[6] Barlow J, Pocock W. The significance of late systolic murmurs and mid-late systolic clicks. *Am Heart J* 1963; 66: 443.

[7] Mills WR, Barber JE, Ratliff NB, Cosgrove DM III, Vesely I, Griffin BP. Biomechanical and echocardiographic characterization of flail mitral leaflet due to myxomatous disease: further evidence for early surgical intervention. *Am Heart J* 2004; 148: 144–50.

[8] Grande-Allen KJ, Griffin BP, Ratliff NB, Cosgrove DM, Vesely I. Glycosaminoglycan profiles of myxomatous mitral leaflets and chordae parallel the severity of mechanical alterations. *J Am Coll Cardiol* 2003; 42: 271–77.

[9] Trochu JN, Kyndt F, Schott JJ, et al. Clinical characteristics of a familial inherited myxomatous valvular dystrophy mapped to Xq28. *J Am Coll Cardiol* 2000; 35: 1890–97.

[10] Bursi F, Enriquez-Sarano M, Jacobsen SJ, Roger VL. Mitral regurgitation after myocardial infarction: a review. *Am J Med* 2006; 119: 103–120.

[11] Grose R, Strain J, Cohen MV. Pulmonary arterial V waves in mitral regurgitation: clinical and experimental observations. *Circulation* 1984; 69: 214–22.

[12] Yoran C, Yellin EL, Becker R, Gabbay S, Frater RW, Sonnenblick EH. Dynamic aspects of acute mitral regurgitation: effects of ventricular volume, pressure and contractility on the effective regurgitant orifice area. *Circulation* 1979; 60: 170–76.

[13] Schwammenthal E, Chen C, Benning F, Block M, Breithardt G, Levine R. Dynamics of mitral regurgitant flow and orifice area. Physiologic application of the proximal flow convergence method: clinical data and experimental testing. *Circulation* 1994; 90: 307–22.

[14] Keren G, Bier A, Strom J, Laniado S, Sonnenblick E, LeJemtel T. Dynamics of mitral regurgitation during nitroglycerin therapy: a Doppler echocardiographic study. *Am Heart J* 1986; 112: 517–25.

[15] Lebrun F, Lancellotti P, Pierard LA. Quantitation of functional mitral regurgitation during bicycle exercise in patients with heart failure. *J Am Coll Cardiol* 2001; 38: 1685–92.

[16] Enriquez-Sarano M, Basmadjian A, Rossi A, Bailey K, Seward J, Tajik A. Progression of mitral regurgitation: a prospective Doppler echocardiographic study. *J Am Coll Cardiol* 1999; 34: 1137–44.

[17] Starling MR, Kirsch MM, Montgomery DG, Gross MD. Impaired left ventricular contractile function in patients with long-term mitral regurgitation and normal ejection fraction. *J Am Coll Cardiol* 1993; 22: 239–50.

[18] Enriquez-Sarano M, Tajik A, Schaff H, et al. Echocardiographic prediction of left ventricular function after correction of mitral regurgitation: results and clinical implications. *J Am Coll Cardiol* 1994; 24: 1536–43.

[19] Matsumura T, Ohtaki E, Tanaka K, et al. Echocardiographic prediction of left ventricular dysfunction after mitral valve repair for mitral regurgitation as an indicator to decide the optimal timing of repair. *J Am Coll Cardiol* 2003; 42: 458–63.

[20] Messika-Zeitoun D, Johnson BD, Nkomo V, et al. Cardiopulmonary exercise testing determination of functional capacity in mitral regurgitation: physiologic and outcome implications. *J Am Coll Cardiol* 2006; 47: 2521–27.

[21] Freeman W, Schaff H, Khanderia B, et al. Intraoperative evaluation of mitral valve regurgitation and repair by transesophageal echocardiography: incidence and significance of systolic anterior motion. *J Am Coll Cardiol* 1992; 20: 599–609.

[22] Zoghbi WA, Enriquez-Sarano M, Foster E, et al. Evaluation of the severity of native valvular regurgitation with two-dimensional and Doppler echocardiography: a report from the Task Force on Valvular Regurgitation of the American Society of Echocardiography. *J Am Soc Echocardiogr* 2003; 16: 777–802.

[23] Enriquez-Sarano M, Tajik A, Bailey K, Seward J. Color flow imaging compared with quantitative doppler assessment of severity of mitral regurgitation: influence of eccentricity of jet and mechanism of regurgitation. *J Am Coll Cardiol* 1993; 21: 1211–19.

[24] Enriquez-Sarano M, Bailey K, Seward J, Tajik A, Krohn M, Mays J. Quantitative Doppler assessment of valvular regurgitation. *Circulation* 1993; 87: 841–48.

[25] Enriquez-Sarano M, Miller FAJ, Hayes SN, Bailey KR, Tajik AJ, Seward JB. Effective mitral regurgitant orifice area: clinical use and pitfalls of the proximal isovelocity surface area method. *J Am Coll Cardiol* 1995; 25: 703–09.

[26] Lang RM, Bierig M, Devereux RB, et al. Recommendations for chamber quantification: a report from the American Society of Echocardiography's Guidelines and Standards Committee and the

Chamber Quantification Writing Group, developed in conjunction with the European Association of Echocardiography, a branch of the European Society of Cardiology. *J Am Soc Echocardiogr* 2005; 18: 1440–63.

[27] Thomas JD. Howleaky is that mitral valve? Simplified Doppler methods to measure regurgitant orifice area. *Circulation* 1997;95 (3):548–50.

[28] Leung D, Griffi n B, Stewart W, Cosgrove D, Thomas J, Marwick T. Left Ventricular function after valve repair for chronic mitral regurgitation: predictive value of preoperative assessment of contractile reserve by exercise echocardiography. *J Am Coll Cardiol* 1996; 28: 1198–205.

[29] Horstkotte D, Loogen F, Kleikamp G, Schulte HD, Trampisch HJ, Bircks W. The infl uence of heart valve replacement on the natural history of isolated mitral, aortic and multivalvular disease. *Z Kardiol* 1983; 72: 494–503.

[30] Ling H, Enriquez-Sarano M, Seward J, et al. Clinical outcome of mitral regurgitation due to flail leaflets. *N Eng J Med* 1996; 335: 1417–23.

[31] Grigioni F, Enriquez-Sarano M, Ling L, et al. Sudden death in mitral regurgitation due to flail leaflet. *J Am Coll Cardiol* 1999; 34: 2078–85.

[32] Kligfield P, Hochreiter C, Niles N, Devereux R, Borer J. Relation of sudden death in pure mitral regurgitation, with and without mitral valve prolapse, to repetitive ventricular arrhythmias and right and left ventricular ejection fractions. *Am J Cardiol* 1987; 60: 397–99.

[33] Rosenhek R, Rader F, Klaar U, et al. Outcome of watchful waiting in asymptomatic severe mitral regurgitation. *Circulation* 2006; 113: 2238–44.

[34] Enriquez-Sarano M, Avierinos JF, Messika-Zeitoun D, et al. Quantitative determinants of the outcome of asymptomatic mitral regurgitation. *N Engl J Med* 2005; 352: 875–83.

[35] 68) Grigioni F, Avierinos JF, Ling LH, et al. Atrial fibrillation complicating the course of degenerative mitral regurgitation. Determinants and long-term outcome. *J Am Coll Cardiol* 2002; 40: 84–92.

[36] Avierinos JF, Brown RD, Foley DA, et al. Cerebral ischemic events after diagnosis of mitral valve prolapse: a community-based study of incidence and predictive factors. *Stroke* 2003; 34: 1339–44.

[37] Hochreiter C, Niles N, Devereux R, Kligfi eld P, Borer J. Mitral regurgitation: relationship of noninvasive descriptors of right and left ventricular performance to clinical and hemodynamic findings and to

prognosis in medically and surgically treated patients. *Circulation* 1986; 73: 900–12.

[38] Detaint D, Sundt TM, Nkomo VT, et al. Surgical correction of mitral regurgitation in the elderly: outcomes and recent improvements. *Circulation* 2006; 114: 265–72.

[39] Tribouilloy C, Enriquez-Sarano M, Schaff H, et al. Impact of preoperative symptoms on survival after surgical correction of organic mitral regurgitation: rationale for optimizing surgical indications. Circulation 1999; 99: 400–05.

[40] Shuhaiber J, Anderson RJ. Meta-analysis of clinical outcomes following surgical mitral valve repair or replacement. *Eur J Cardiothorac Surg* 2007; 31: 267–75.

[41] Tribouilloy C, Enriquez-Sarano M, Schaff H, et al. Excess mortality due to coronary artery disease after valvular surgery: secular trends in valvular regurgitation and effect of internal mammary bypass. *Circulation* 1998; 98: II108–15.

[42] David TE, Ivanov J, Armstrong S, Rakowski H. Late outcomes of mitral valve repair for floppy valves: implications for asymptomatic patients. *J Thorac Cardiovasc Surg* 2003; 125: 1143–52.

[43] Crawford MH, Souchek J, Oprian CA, Miller DC, Rahimtoola S, Giacomini JC, Sethi G, Hammermeister KE. Determinants of survival and left ventricular performance after mitral valve replacement. Department of Veterans Affairs Cooperative Study on Valvular Heart Disease. *Circulation* 1990;81 (4):1173–81.

[44] Yun KL, Sintek CF, Miller DC, et al. Randomized trial of partial versus complete chordal preservation methods of mitral valve replacement: A preliminary report. *Circulation* 1999; 100 (19 suppl): II90–94.

[45] Enriquez-Sarano M, Schaff H, Orszulak T, Bailey K, Tajik A, Frye R. Congestive heart failure after surgical correction of mitral regurgitation. A long-term study. *Circulation* 1995; 92: 2496–503.

[46] Delahaye JP, Gare JP, Viguier E, Delahaye F, De Gevigney G, Milon H. Natural history of severe mitral regurgitation. *Eur Heart J* 1991; (12 Suppl B):5–9.

[47] Ling LH, Enriquez-Sarano M, Seward JB, Tajik AJ, Schaff HV, Bailey KR, Frye RL. Clinical outcome of mitral regurgitation due to flail leaflet. *N Engl J Med* 1996;335 (19):1417–23.

[48] Tishler M, Rowan M, LeWinter M. Effect of Enalapril on left ventricular mass and volumes in asymptomatic chronic, severe mitral

regurgitation secondary to mitral valve prolapse. *Am J Cardiol.* 1998; 82: 242–45.

[49] Levine H, Gaasch W. Vasoactive drugs in chronic regurgitant lesions of the mitral and aortic valves. *J Am Coll Cardiol* 1996; 28: 1083–91.

[50] Schon H. Hemodynamic and morphologic changes after long-term angiotensin converting enzyme inhibition in patients with chronic valvular regurgitation. *J Hypertens* 1994; 12: S95–104.

[51] Dujardin KS, Enriquez-Sarano M, Bailey KR, Seward JB, Tajik AJ. Effect of losartan on degree of mitral regurgitation quantified by echocardiography. *Am J Cardiol* 2001; 87: 570–76.

[52] Nagatsu M, Spinale FG, Koide M, et al. Bradycardia and the role of beta-blockade in the amelioration of left ventricular dysfunction. *Circulation* 2000; 101: 653–59.

[53] Bonow RO, Carabello BA, Kanu C, de Leon Jr AC, Faxon DP, Freed MD, GaaschWH, Lytle BW, Nishimura RA, O'Gara PT, O'Rourke RA, Otto CM, Shah PM, Shanewise JS, Smith Jr SC, Jacobs AK, Adams CD, Anderson JL, Antman EM, Faxon DP, Fuster V, Halperin JL, Hiratzka LF, Hunt SA, Lytle BW, Nishimura R, Page RL, Riegel B. ACC/AHA 2006 guidelines for the management of patients with valvular heart disease: a report of the American College of Cardiology/American Heart Association Task Force on Practice Guidelines (writing committee to revise the 1998 Guidelines for the Management of Patients With Valvular Heart Disease): developed in collaboration with the Society of Cardiovascular Anesthesiologists: endorsed by the Society for Cardiovascular Angiography and Interventions and the Society of Thoracic Surgeons. *Circulation* 2006; 114 (5):e84–231.

[54] Enriquez-Sarano M, Tajik A, Schaff H, Orszulak T, Bailey K, Frye R. Echocardiographic prediction of survival after surgical correction of organic mitral regurgitation. *Circulation* 1994; 90: 830–37.

[55] Sherrid MV, Clark RD, Cohn K. Echocardiographic analysis of left atrial size before and after operation in mitral valve disease. *Am J Cardiol* 1979;43 (2):171–8.

[56] Raanani E, Albage A, David TE, Yau TM, Armstrong S. The efficacy of the Cox/maze procedure combined with mitral valve surgery: a matched control study. *Eur J Cardiothorac Surg* 2001;19 (4):438–42.

[57] Nashef SA, Roques F, Michel P, Gauducheau E, Lemeshow S, Salamon R. European system for cardiac operative risk evaluation (EuroSCORE). *Eur J Cardiothorac Surg* 1999;16 (1):9–13.

[58] Grossi EA, Goldberg JD, LaPietra A, Ye X, Zakow P, Sussman M, Delianides J, Culliford AT, Esposito RA, Ribakove GH, Galloway AC, Colvin SB. Ischemic mitral valve reconstruction and replacement: comparison of long-term survival and complications. *J Thorac Cardiovasc Surg* 2001; 122 (6):1107–24.
[59] Seeburger J, Borger MA, Falk V, Kuntze T, Czesla M, Walther T, Doll N, Mohr FW. Minimal invasive mitral valve repair for mitral regurgitation: results of 1339 consecutive patients. *Euro J Cardiothorac Surg* 2008.
[60] Executive Summary STS Spring 2006 Report: *The Society of Thoracic Surgery;* 2006.
[61] Braunberger E, Deloche A, Berrebi A, Abdallah F, Celestin JA, Meimoun P, Chatellier G, Chauvaud S, Fabiani JN, Carpentier A. Very long-term results (more than 20 years) of valve repair with Carpentier's techniques in non-rheumatic mitral valve insufficiency. *Circulation* 2001;104[suppl I]I:I-8-I-11.
[62] Gillinov AM. Cosgrove DM III. Modified sliding leaflet technique for repair of the mitral valve. *Ann Thorac Surg* 1999;68:2356-7.
[63] Mutimedia Mannual of Cardiothoracic Surgery. Patrick Perier. Quadrangular resection for repair of posterior leaflet prolapse. 2005.
[64] Gazoni LM, Fedoruk LM, Kern JA, Dent JM, Reece TB, Tribble CG, Smith PW, Lisle TC, Kron IL. A simplified approach to degenerative disease: triangular resections of the mitral valve. *Ann Thorac Surg* 2007;83:1658-65.
[65] Brown ML, Abel MD, Click RL, Morford RG, Dearani JA, Sundt TM, Orszulak TA, Schaff HV. Systolic anterior motion after mitral valve repair: Is surgical intervention necessary? *J Thorac Cardiovasc Surg* 2007;133:136-43.
[66] Calafiore AM, Di Mauro M, Iaco AL, Mazzei V, Teodori G, Gallina S, Weltert L, Samoun M, Di Giammarco G. Overreduction of the posterior annulus in surgical treatment of degenerative mitral regurgitation. *Ann Thorac Surg* 2006;81:1310-6.
[67] Von Oppel UO, Mohr FW. Chordal replacement for both minimally invasive and conventional mitral valve surgery using premeasured Gore-Tex loops. *Ann Thorac Surg* 2000;70:2166-8.
[68] Gillinov AM, Banbury MK. Pre-measured artificial chordae for mitral valve repair. *Ann Thorac Surg* 2007;84:2127-9.
[69] Gillinov AM, Cosgrove DM III. Chordal transfer for repair of anterior leaflet prolapse. *Semin Thorac Cardiovasc Surg* 2004;16:169-73.

[70] Lapenna E, Torracca L, De Bonis M, La Canna G, Crescenzi G, Alferi O. Minimally invasive mitral valve repair in the context of Barlow's disease. *Ann Thorac Surg* 2005;79:1496-9.

[71] Bhudia SK, McCarthy PM, Smedira NG: Edge-to-edge (Alfieri) mitral repair: Results in diverse clinical settings. *Ann Thorac Surg* 2004; 77:1598.[Abstract/Free Full Text].

[72] Maslow AD, Regan MM, Haering JM, et al: Echocardiographic predictors of left ventricular outflow tract obstruction and systolic anterior motion of the mitral valve after mitral valve reconstruction for myxomatous valve disease. *J Am Coll Cardiol* 1999; 34:2096. [Abstract/Free Full Text].

[73] Gillinov AM, Shortt KG, Cosgrove DM III. Commissural closure for repair of mitral commissural prolapse. *Ann Thorac Surg* 2005;80:1135-6.

[74] Savage EB, Ferguson TB Jr., DiSesa VJ: Use of mitral valve repair: Analysis of contemporary United States experience reported to the Society of Thoracic Surgeons National Cardiac Database. *Ann Thorac Surg* 2003; 75:820.[Abstract/Free Full Text].

[75] Gillinov AM, Cosgrove DM, Shiota T, et al: Cosgrove-Edwards annuloplasty system: Midterm results. *Ann Thorac Surg* 2000; 69:717.[Abstract/Free FullText].

[76] Carpentier A: Cardiac valve surgery: The "French correction." *J Thorac Cardiovasc Surg* 1983; 86:323.[Medline].

[77] Shuhaiber J, Anderson RJ. Meta-analysis of clinical outcomes following surgical mitral valve repair or replacement. *Eur J Cardiothorac Surg* 2007;31:267-75.

[78] David TE, Ivanov J, Armstrong S, Rakowski H. Late outcomes of mitral valve repair for floppy valves: implications for asymptomatic patients. *J Thorac Cardiovasc Surg* 2003;125:1143-52.

[79] Russo A, Grigioni F, Avierinos JF, et al. Thromboembolic complications after surgical correction of mitral regurgitation incidence, predictors, and clinical implications. *J Am Coll Cardiol* 2008;51: 1203-11.

[80] Mohty D, Orszulak TA, Schaff HV, Avierinos JF, Tajik JA, Enriquez-Sarano M. Very long-term survival and durability of mitral valve repair for mitral valve prolapse. *Circulation* 2001;104:Suppl 1:I-1–I-7.

[81] Smedira NG, Selman R, Cosgrove DM, McCarthy PM, Lytle BW, Taylor PC, Apperson-Hansen C, Stewart RW, Loop FD. Repair of

anterior leaflet prolapse: Chordal transfer is superior to chordal shortening. *J Thorac Cardiovasc Surg*1996;112:287-292.

[82] Mihaljevic T, Jarrett CM, Gillinov AM, Williams SJ, DeVilliers PA, Stewart WJ, Svensson LG, Sabik, III JF, Blackstone EH. Robotic repair of posterior mitral valve prolapse versus conventional approaches: Potential realized. *J Thorac Cardiovasc Surg* 2011;141:72-80.

[83] Alfieri O, Maisano F, De Bonis M, et al. The double-orifice technique in mitral valve repair: a simple solution for complex problems. *J Thorac Cardiovasc Surg* 2001; 122: 674–81.

[84] Feldman T, Wasserman HS, Herrmann HC, et al. Percutaneous mitral valve repair using the edge-to-edge technique: six-month results of the EVEREST phase I clinical trial. *J Am Coll Cardiol* 2005; 46: 2134–40.

[85] Byrne MJ, Kaye DM, Mathis M, Reuter DG, Alferness CA, Power JM. Percutaneous mitral annular reduction provides continued benefit in an ovine model of dilated cardiomyopathy. *Circulation* 2004; 110: 3088–92.

[86] Webb JG, Harnek J, Munt BI, et al. Percutaneous transvenous mitral annuloplasty: initial human experience with device implantation in the coronary sinus. *Circulation* 2006; 113: 851–55.

In: Mitral Valve Disease
Editor: Richard R. Heuser
ISBN: 978-1-61942-309-1

Chapter 2

ISCHEMIC MITRAL REGURGITATION

***Turki B. Albacker*[1] *and Benoit De Varrennes*[2]**
[1]Assistant Professor, Department of Cardiac Surgery, King Fahad Cardiac Center, King Khalid Medical City, King Saud University, Riyadh, Saudi Arabia
[2]Associate Professor, Chairman of Department of Cardiac Surgery, McGill University Heath Center McGill University, Montreal, Canada

ABSTRACT

Ischemic mitral regurgitation (IMR) is present in 10%-20% of patients with Coronary Artery Disease (CAD) and is associated with a markedly worse prognosis and long-term patient survival in comparison with other types of mitral regurgitation. IMR can be classified into an acute type and a chronic type. Acute IMR occurs as a result of papillary muscle rupture complicating acute myocardial infarction or as a result of acute ischemic episodes involving the Left circumflex or right coronary Artery, resulting in 'Flash pulmonary edema'. Chronic IMR is primarily a ventricular problem, not a valvular problem, caused by LV remodeling resulting from ischemic cardiomyopathy. Chronic IMR is characterizes by a dynamic nature that may affect the degree of regurgitation and is related to several factor, including LV function and loading conditions. The majority of patients with chronic IMR is asymptomatic and may be incidentally discovered during evaluation for myocardial revasculari-zation. Less commonly, those patients may present with progressive heart failure when MR is moderate to severe. Transthoracic /Transesophageal Echocardiography represents the gold standard for evaluation if IMR. It has been used to establish the diagnosis of IMR as well as to quantify the degree of regurgitation and to identify the underlying mechanism of valve dysfunction to guide any possible therapy. Cardiac MRI has recently emerged as single-pass diagnostic tool that allows evaluation of valvular/ subvalvular and LV geometry, along with myocardial viability, which has recently been shown to be predictive of post-revascularization outcome on IMR. Ischemic Mitral Regurgitation (IMR) continues to be a perplexing clinical problem and controversy continues with regards to optimal therapeutic modality. We review in this chapter different diagnostic and therapeutic modalities for chronic IMR with emphasis on the decision making process supported by up to date review of the available evidence.

INTRODUCTION

Ischemic mitral regurgitation (IMR) is the regurgitation seen with structurally normal valve leaflets that occurs in approximately 20% of patients after myocardial infarction (MI) and 56% of patients with congestive heart failure (CHF) caused by ischemic cardiomyopathy [1]. The initiating event is an ischemic insult that results in remodeling of the LV toward a more spherical shape and new wall motion abnormalities. These changes lead to annular dilation and subvalvular distortion that prevent the mitral leaflets from coapting and closing completely during the contraction phase. Mitral regurgitation (MR) consists of systolic retrograde flow from the left ventricle (LV) to the left atrium (LA) because of the lack of adequate coaptation of the leaflets and a pressure gradient between the two cavities. Appropriate systolic coaptation of the anterior and posterior mitral leaflets depends on normal anatomy and function of the different components of the mitral valve apparatus: annulus, leaflets, chordae, papillary muscles, and the LV wall. Ischaemic MR does not necessarily imply the presence of true myocardial ischaemia. This term is used to describe the clinical entity of chronic coronary artery disease (CAD) with frequently a prior history of one or more MI, which induced progressive LV global or regional pathological remodeling, usually in the absence of reversible ischaemia [2].

Definition and Classification

IMR is defined as mitral regurgitation that results from one or more LV segmental wall motion abnormalities as a consequence of significant CAD in the territory supplying the wall motion abnormality. The mitral valve leaflets and chordae tendineae are structurally normal [3].

IMR can be classified into acute and chronic. Acute IMR occurs within two weeks of the acute MI as a result of the rupture of a papillary muscle, most frequently a head of a posteromedial papillary muscle. This condition is associated with a very high mortality rate in the absence of immediate surgical intervention. Surgery, most often valve replacement, is warranted after stabilization of the haemodynamic status using an intra-aortic balloon pump and vasodilators [4]. Its incidence and clinical importance are largely under estimated, partly because physical examination is rather insensitive. Prompt in-hospital revascularization can prevent or reverse acute IMR [5], reduce localized LV remodeling and chronic IMR [6] and increases survival in patients with acute IMR presenting with shock [7].

Acute IMR could also occur without rupture of the papillary muscle secondary to an active ischaemic episode. It is clinically referred to as a ''flash pulmonary oedema''[8]. It is linked to the presence of a significant stenosis of the right or left circumflex coronary artery. In this situation, the primary treatment is to prevent the episodes of active myocardial ischaemia by a revascularization procedure.

Chronic IMR occurs more than two weeks after the acute ischemic as a result of segmental or global ventricular dysfunction. It results from an imbalance between tethering forces (annular dilatation, LV dilatation, papillary muscles displacement, LV sphericity) and closing forces (reduction of LV contractility, global LV dyssynchrony, papillary muscle dyssynchrony, altered mitral systolic annular contraction) [2]. Chronic IMR results, in 95% of cases, from a type IIIb dysfunction (restricted leaflet motion). It is important to note that in the remaining 5%, an ischaemic elongation of the papillary muscle may cause prolapse in the corresponding area (type II dysfunction). Chronic IMR is characteristically dynamic during exercise and its increased severity during exercise identifies a subgroup of patients at higher risk of cardiac events [8].

PATHOPHYSIOLOGY

In IMR, the initiating event is an ischemic insult to the ventricular wall and the subvalvular apparatus attached to it. This insult results in new wall motion abnormalities and LV remodeling toward a spherical shape. These changes lead to annular dilation and subvalvular distortion (ie, papillary muscle displacement and tethered chordae). Because the mitral leaflets are tethered to a fixed maximal distance by the papillary muscle and chordae, remodeling prevents the leaflets from coapting and closing completely during the contraction phase. Additionally, new wall motion abnormalities may prevent the production of sufficient ventricular closing force to oppose the tethering and the closure of the leaflets. The variations in MR and effective regurgitant orifice are determined by the balance of the forces that act on the mitral leaflets: the tethering forces and the closing forces [9]. The regurgitation peaks in early systole, decreases during mid-systole, and peaks again in late systole [10, 11]. The paradoxical decrease in mid-systolic regurgitation occurs because in mid-systole, peak LV pressure maximizes leaflet closure [12]. The volume overload due to MR contributes to a vicious circle: the more remodeled LV, the more severe MR which leads to further LV dilatation and thus, further MR. This cycle has important effects on LV geometry with spherical transformation. Although MR reduces impedance and has an unloading effect, the LV dilatation increases ventricular wall stress leading to worsened LV compliance. This in turn leads to increased LA pressure and pulmonary arterial hypertension.

The presence of IMR is associated with increased morbidity and mortality. When compared with patients without MR, the patients with acute MI and MR are older, more frequently female, have more frequently a history of previous MI and a more severe CAD. Many studies have shown that IMR is an independent predictor of cardiovascular death [13, 14]. The relative risk varies from 1.48 to 7.5. Among one-month survivors of MI, a community study has showed that the presence of IMR is associated with a three-fold increase in the risk of heart failure and a 1.6-fold increased risk of death at 5-year follow-up, independent of LV ejection fraction, Killip class, age and gender [3]. The increased mortality risk relates to the quantified degree of MR [15]. Aronson et al. [16] prospectively studied 1190 patients who had sustained acute MI between 2001 and 2005 stratified according to degree of MR. Within 3 years, 30% of those with moderate or severe regurgitation had been hospitalized for heart failure, compared with 5% of those with no regurgitation. The mortality rates were also substantially higher in those with moderate or severe regurgitation (35% at 3 years; hazard ratio [HR], 5.5; 95% CI, 2.3–9.1) compared with those with no regurgitation (8% at 3 years). Of note was that even mild regurgitation was a risk factor for midterm mortality (HR, 2.0; 95% CI, 1.4–3.0).

Currently there are no studies of outcome using sophisticated measures of LV function to determine whether IMR is a predictor of outcome independent of the amount of LV dysfunction present. Supporting this concept is the lack of evidence that correction of IMR prolongs life, which would be expected to occur if MR were an independent risk factor for death beyond the LV dysfunction present. The dynamic component of IMR has also prognostic implications. At 3-year follow-up, there is a five-fold increase in the relative risk of death in patients with an exercise-induced increase of ≥13 mm2 of the ERO area 17. The multivariate analysis shows that severe MR at rest (≥20 mm2) is also an independent predictor of death. The severity of MR at rest has, in contrast, no independent value to predict cardiovascular morbidity and in particular hospitalization for cardiac decompensation. The dynamic component is the best predictor of such complications. In 20% of patients, an improvement in the severity of IMR is observed during exercise. These patients have a better long-term prognosis [17]. Such a reduction is most frequently observed in patients with contractile reserve, especially of the posterior wall, resulting in a temporary reduced distortion of the mitral valve [18].

ASSESSMENT

Echocardiography

Quantification of Ischaemic Mitral Regurgitation

The quantitative methods include the Doppler volumetric method that measures the stroke volume through both mitral and aortic valves. The regurgitant volume is then calculated as the difference between these two stroke volumes. The flow-convergence method is more practical and permits the measurement of effective regurgitant orifice (ERO) area and regurgitant volume (RV). These parameters are calculated from the measured proximal isovelocity surface area (PISA). A number of factors have to be considered when measuring the PISA. The PISA radius should not be measured at only one time point, but averaged through systole because of the radius variations during systole. The flow convergence should be hemispheric to avoid an underestimated calculation of ERO and regurgitant volume [19]. Finally, when several jets are present; several flow-convergence regions can be added but this method has not been validated. In this condition, the most reliable calculation of regurgitant volume and ERO area would be averaging the measurements from the quantitative Doppler and the PISA methods.

Assessment of Mitral Leaflets and Subvalvular Apparatus

These include leaflet length, tenting area, apical displacement of the coaptation point, distance between the posterior papillary muscle head and the intervalvular fibrosa, lateral and posterior displacement of the papillary muscles and leaflet angles. The direction of the regurgitant jet helps characterizing the symmetry/asymmetry of the MV distortion.

The application of 3D echocardiography has improved our ability to localize and quantify tethering and allows us to assess volumes and areas rather than single measures of distance, as in 2D echocardiography. In assessing the degree of leaflet tethering, 3D echocardiography has an advantage in that it considers the entire valve and is independent of the plane of selection, asymmetry of tenting, and annular dilatation [20]. Using 3D echocardiography in an ovine model, Ryan et al. [21] described methods that allow comprehensive analysis of tethering of the entire valve; using this technique, they produced data suggesting that tenting and valve remodeling may be more widespread than is appreciated on 2D echocardiography and may not be as limited to the posterior annulus as generally assumed.

Left Ventricular Function and Geometry

Since IMR is a ventricular disease, LV assessment is an essential part of the workup. This will include LV ejection fraction, wall motion abnormalities and myocardial thickness, measuring end-diastolic and end-systolic volumes and finally assessment of sphericity. These parameters are highly dependent on loading conditions. The mitral closing force can be estimated by the measurement of intra LV dyssynchrony and the non-invasive calculation of LV maximal dP/dt, obtainable by the continuous-wave Doppler method. Left ventricular dP/dt is calculated by the simplified Bernouilli equation. It is important to recognize that dP/dt is an isovolumetric measure of LV function. Because no true isovolumic phase exists in MR (ejection occurs into the LA well before the aortic valve opens) dP/dt not only varies directly with contractility but also inversely with the severity of the MR present.

Exercise Echocardiography

Exercise testing is very helpful to detect the dynamic nature of the IMR and it is especially important in asymptomatic patients or those with mild symptoms for early detection and management before irreversible changes occur in the ventricle. The exercise echocardiogram is performed on a dedicated table, in semi-supine position, and several numerous parameters can be obtained during exercise as well as during the recovery period [22]. These include ERO area, RV, trans-tricuspid pressure gradient and systolic pulmonary artery pressure. Other interesting measurements can be obtained during exercise like the tenting area (its changes correlate well with changes in the severity of MR) and LV dys-synchrony (exercise-induced increase of dys-synchrony correlates with increased severity of MR and reduction in stroke volume during exercise) [23].

Cardiac Catheterization

Coronary angiography and left heart catheterization are essential for assessment of patients with IMR. All of those patients will require coronary bypass at the time of mitral valve operation. Patients with poor targets, diffusely small and diseased coronaries and LV dysfunction might be better suited for heart transplant. Right heart catheterization is helpful in patients with pulmonary hypertension to estimate how much is contributed by the left sided lesion through measuring pulmonary capillary wedge pressure (PCWP).

Cardiac Magnetic Resonance Imaging (MRI)

Magnetic resonance imaging is a unique tool that gives the clinician a comprehensive assessment of all relevant features of ischemic cardio-myopathy: ventricular function and size, myocardial scarring, and severity of MR [24].

Assessment of Myocardial Viability

Myocardial viability may have an important role in selecting patients with IMR who may benefit from revascularization alone with out mitral intervention. Penicka and his colleagues [25] showed that surgical revascularization in these patients with a mild form of ischemic cardiomyopathy resulted in decreased MR, reversal in left ventricular remodeling, and improved survival. The absence of viability or presence of ventricular dys-synchrony is indicative of advanced-stage ischemic cardiomyopathy in which recovery from IMR with isolated coronary artery bypass grafting (CABG) is unlikely. In these patients, concomitant mitral valve repair (MVr) should be considered.

MANAGEMENT

Medical Treatment

Medical treatment is considered the first line of treatment. It delays the need for surgical intervention while controlling the patient symptoms, preventing myocardial ischemia and delaying ventricular remodeling. It also helps in preoperative optimization in patients in whom surgical therapy is indicated. However, there is no evidence that medical therapy has any effect on survival. Medical treatment includes preload reduction using diuretics and nitrates, B-blockers to decrease the heart rate and consequently decrease myocardial oxygen consumption and after load reduction using angiotensin converting enzyme (ACE) inhibitors to decrease the RV.

Surgical Treatment

In severe MR secondary to acute MI, the cause of the MR should be established, because the MR may be due to a ruptured papillary muscle, papillary muscle displacement with leaflet tethering, or annular dilatation from severe LV dilatation. Those patients with an acute rupture of the papillary muscle should undergo surgery on an emergency basis, with either MVr or MV replacement (MVR) [26]. In those patients with papillary muscle dysfunction, treatment should initially consist of hemodynamic stabilization, usually with insertion of an intra-aortic balloon pump (IABP). Surgery should be considered for those patients who do not improve with aggressive medical therapy. Correction of acute severe IMR usually requires valve surgery in addition to revascularization. CABG alone may improve LV function and reduce ischemic MR in selected patients with chronic IMR [27], especially those with transient severe MR due to ischemia, in whom myocardial revass-cularization can eliminate episodes of severe MR. However, CABG alone is usually insufficient and leaves many patients with significant residual MR, and these patients would benefit from concomitant MV surgery at the time of the CABG [28-30]. The indication for MV operation in the patient who undergoes CABG with mild to moderate MR is still unclear, but there are data to indicate benefit of MVr in such patients [31]. In symptomatic patients with severe IMR and no option for revascularization, MVr may be considered. However, when the LV function is severely impaired, surgery is more likely to be considered if myocardial viability is present, if comorbidity is low, if IMR increases dynamically during exercise, if the LV is not severely remodeled, and if the revascularization can be almost complete. In the other cases, cardiac transplantation remains the preferable approach since it is associated with a better 5-year outcome. Very ill patients should be treated conservatively with revascularisation alone [32]. Low risk patients can be further stratified with exercise echocardiography [33]. Patients with a dynamic increase in IMR (ERO >13 mm2) during exercise might be submitted for combined surgery, while patients with either no significant changes or exercise induced reduction in IMR as a result of recruitable function in the inferobasal wall might be referred for CABG alone.

Indications for Surgical Intervention

Symptomatic Patients

Symptomatic patients with severe IMR should have MVr provided that ventricular function is preserved (E.F >30%) (class I). When there is severe LV dysfunction (E.F < 30%), surgery might be considered if the patient is symptomatic and revascularization is possible (class IIa). In these setting MVr could be considered but MVR with chordal preservation is a reasonable and safe option. If revascularization is not an option in patients with severe LV dysfunction, patient should be considered for heart transplantation or optimal medical therapy if not a candidate for transplant.

Asymptomatic Patients:

*A*symptomatic patients with severe IMR should be considered for MV surgery if there is any impairment of ventricular function (E.F < 60%) or evidence of ventricular remodeling (ESD < 55 mm) (class IIa). MV surgery could also be considered in asymptomatic patients with new onset atrial fibrillation or with pulmonary hypertension (class IIb).

Moderate IMR

Patients with moderate IMR might be considered for MV surgery when revascularization is indicated and feasible (class IIa). If revascularization is not possible, then it becomes controversial whether MV surgery should be performed or not and the decision should be made on patient-to-patient bases.

Surgical Options

A) Mitral Valve Repair

Restrictive Annuloplasty

The most common type of surgery performed for ischemic MR is an undersized mitral annuloplasty. In this technique, a small (size 24 to 26 mm) mitral annuloplasty ring is used, which causes a reduction in the antero-posterior (septolateral) diameter of the MV increasing the surface of coaptation. The procedure is fairly easy to perform and reproducible. Over the past few years, many different types of prosthetic rings have been developed, some are flexible, others rigid, some are complete, others incomplete. However, there are no definite data that show that one ring is superior to another. The drawback with the undersized annuloplasty technique is the high rate of failure. In an article from Cleveland Clinic, 585 patients who had undersized annuloplasty surgery over a 17-year period were examined [34]. In 28% of the patients, moderate or more MR developed 6 months post-operatively. It is felt that the reason for the recurrent MR is that the underlying process of LV dilatation from LV remodeling continues despite having "fixed" the valve. This remodeling causes further tethering of the papillary muscles, especially the posteromedial papillary muscle, and causes the recurrence of MR [35]. Braun et al. [36] recently reported on midterm outcomes of 100 patients who systematically underwent restrictive annuloplasty for IMR. Echocardiography at an average follow-up of 4.3 years showed that 85% of the patients had no or mild MR and the 5-year survival rate was 71%, substantially better than reported in other surgical series. Also observed was a relationship between the preoperative LV end-diastolic diameter (LVEDD) and outcome: patients with an LVEDD ≤ 65 mm had better 5-year survival (80%) and developed sustained LV reverse remodeling compared with patients with an LVEDD greater than 65 mm (5-year survival, 49%; no ventricular reverse remodeling). Although this study shows promising outcomes for patients with IMR and an LVEDD less than 65 mm, it also highlights the need for supplemental or alternative approaches in patients with very dilated ventricles (LVEDD > 65 mm). To address the issue of remodeling, the Carpentier-McCarthy- Adams IMR ETlogix annuloplasty ring was developed. This ring was designed with a reduced middle to medial P2-P3 curvature and a slight dip at the P3-P2 segments to increase coaptation of these tethered segments. Evaluation of this ring in 59 patients showed that after surgery 57 of 59 (97%) patients had grade 0 to 1+ MR, whereas 2 patients had 2+ MR [37]. This new prosthetic ring may improve the durability of MV repair. However, long-term results are not yet available.

Posterior Leaflet Augmentation

Enlarging the mitral leaflet by surgically implanting a pericardial patch represents a novel approach to increasing the coaptation of the mitral leaflets. Langer et al [38] demonstrated the efficacy of the approach in correcting experimental MR and the clinical use of this technique in IMR patients was reported by Devarennes et al [39] in patients with type III IMR. The posterior leaflet is detached at its base from the middle of P2 all the way up to the posterior commissure and then annuloplasty sutures are applied around the circumference of the mitral annulus. A bovine pericardial patch is cut in an oblong fashion with a height of 1 cm and a length of 3.5 to 4.5 cm. The patch was sutured to the edge of the posterior leaflet defect and the posterior mitral annulus with a running 5-0 polytetrafluoroethylene suture (figure 1) The intercommissural distance and the exact surface area of the anterior leaflet were then used to select the appropriate Physio annuloplasty ring. The most common ring size was [28]. It is important to remember that the annuloplasty ring does not need to be undersized when extension of the posterior leaflet is performed. The present approach significantly increases the coaptation surface in the region of the leaflet most affected by tethering from the posteromedial papillary muscle by extending the posterior leaflet height by 1 cm in the area of P3 and the medial half of P2. This also provides a safety margin of tissue in case LV remodeling continues after surgery.

Anterior Leaflet Augmentation

Kincaid et al [40] reported a simple approach to address the tethering of the MV leaflets. The anterior leaflet was augmented in size by creating a defect in it, in the shape of an ellipse. The defect was then filled with a piece of bovine pericardium, and a flexible [27] to 31mm posterior annuloplasty band was placed. This method allowed the level of leaflet coaptation to fall more posteriorly, and towards the level of the displaced papillary muscles (Figure 2).

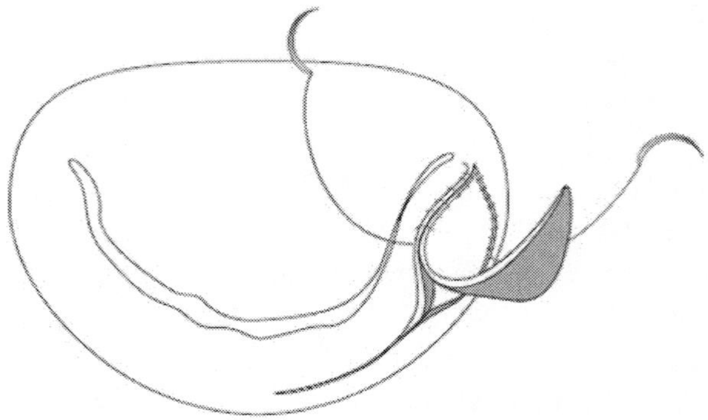

Figure 1. posterior leaflet extension with a bovine pericardial patch.

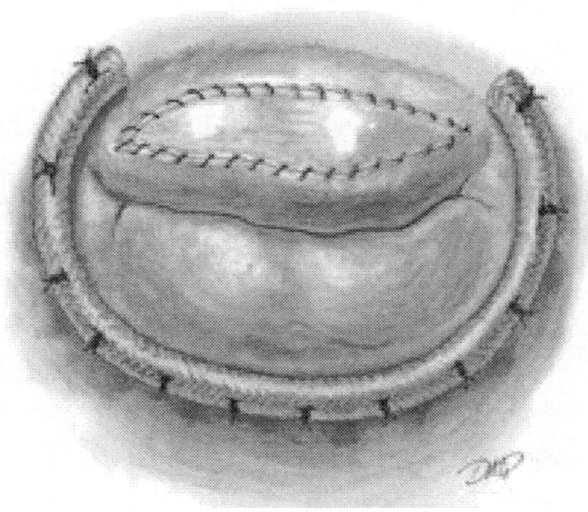

Figure 2. Anterior leaflet extension with a bovine pericardial patch.

Papillary Muscle Repositioning

Attempts to restore a normal anatomic relationship of the papillary muscles may result in less tethering of the leaflets and a potential for more durable elimination of IMR. Animal experiments showed the usefulness of this technique in elimination of leaflet tethering tethering and reduction of regurgitation [41]. In humans, papillary muscle relocation was described by Kron (figure 3) [42]. However, it did not show any difference in long-term outcomes from combining papillary relocation with annuloplasty when compared with annuloplasty alone [43]. Midterm data are awaited on other subvalvular surgical approaches designed to reduce papillary muscle displacement.

Infarct Plication

This procedure is used exclusively in individuals with an inferolateral wall MI. It involves plicating the infarcted region without excision or cardiopulmonary bypass (CPB). This shortens the infarcted area, and brings the displaced papillary muscle back towards the mitral annulus, increasing the zone of coaptation, thus reducing the MR. Ramadan et al [44] used this approach in 3 patients. They placed mattressed sutures over the infarcted region with a Teflon patch. No annuloplasty ring was placed and no bypass was performed to the affected region (Figure 4).

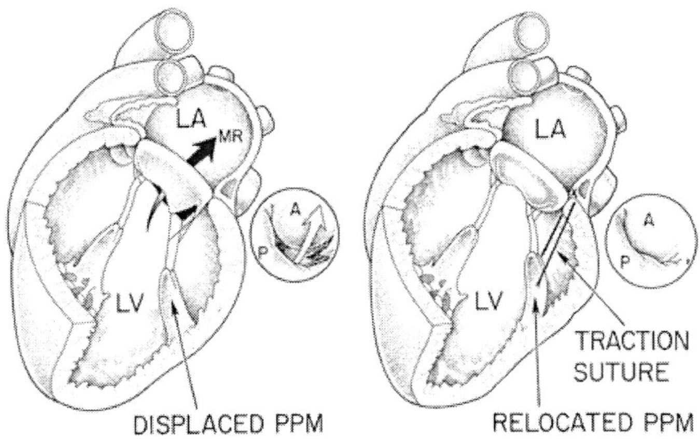

Figure 3. Papillary muscle repositioning.

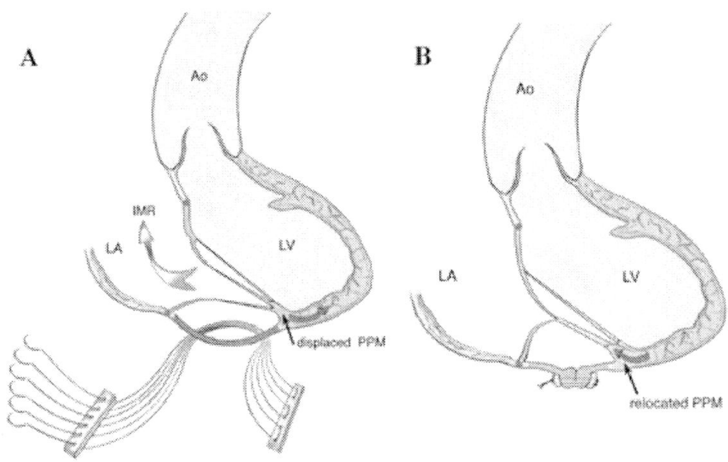

Figure 4. Infarct plication for IMR.

***Division* of Secondary Chordae**

Levine and Schwammenthal 2 previously demonstrated in a series of experiments in sheep that division of secondary MV chordae results in reduced tethering in IMR. Borger et al. [45] reported recently on a series of [43] patients in whom surgeons divided secondary chordae to the anterior leaflet, posterior leaflet, and commissures that arose from the papillary muscle (s) affected by the MI. Additionally, the repair included a moderately undersized (size 26 to 32 mm) flexible, incomplete annuloplasty band. This technique was associated with an improvement in the MV leaflet mobility and less tenting, a reduction in early MR recurrence, without reducing LV function.

***Edge* To Edge Repair**

This technique, also known as the Alfieri stitch, involves placing a suture at the center (A2-P2 portion) of the margins of both leaflets, creating a double orifice MV [46]. An annuloplasty ring needs to be placed with this procedure, because of poor long-term results without it [47]. Even with an annuloplasty ring, the failure rate for this procedure is high. Overall, the edge-to-edge repair has fallen out of favor, and is not frequently used.

B) Mitral Valve Replacement (MVR)

MVr has shown favorable outcomes compared to MVR and it should be tried when ever possible. These recommendations were based on historical data indicating poor outcomes for MVR especially in patients with impaired LV function. The implementation of chordal preservation during MVR and the high rate of recurrence of MR after MVr in patients with advanced ischemic cardiomyopathy lead some groups to advocate MVR in this group of patients [48]. This approach would certainly yield more durable elimination of regurgitation, but it is not clear whether this would offset the incremental risk due to higher surgical mortality, morbidity, and late mortality from valve-related complications. Also, there possibly is a lesser degree of reverse remodeling with MVR compared with MVr. A randomized trial of MVr versus MVR in a high-risk subset of patients with ischemic mitral regurgitation would help clarify the role of MVR. However, contemporary nonrandomized data do not support widespread application of MVR for IMR and suggest that for most patients, the preferred approach is MVr.

C) Other Therapies for Ischemic Cardiomyopathy with Ischemic Mitral Regurgitation

Cardiac Resynchronization Therapy (CRT)

IMR is not by itself an indication for biventricular pacing. It is indicated in patients with IMR who have functional class III– IV despite optimal medical treatment, reduced LV ejection fraction and QRS duration > 0.120 ms especially when a revascularization procedure is not indicated or insufficient to improve the clinical status. The effects of CRT on IMR can be observed acutely or only late after implantation. This treatment is associated with an immediate reduction in the quantified degree of IMR (expected reduction of 35%), which is directly correlated to the improvement in LV systolic performance, increase in LV dP/d and the reduction in the interpapillary muscle activation time delay [49]. Reduction in MR severity also results from a more effective mitral annulus contraction and a significant decrease in systolic tenting area. Thus, in the acute stage, CRT corrects the imbalance between forces acting on the mitral valve and enhances the sphincteric action of the annulus. Besides these acute effects, an additional 10–20% reduction in IMR, that parallels the decrease in LV volumes and the increase in LV dP/dt, occurs some months after CRT. Although this improvement is sustained at 1-year follow-up, it could be attenuated in some patients secondary to the progression of the ischaemic disease [50]. The effect of CRT on dynamic IMR is also progressive and appears in the chronic stage of stimulation. CRT reduces not only IMR at rest but also its dynamic component during exercise. The expected attenuation of exercise induced IMR is about 30% [51]. However, CRT reduces the amount of increase in IMR but does not avoid the development of at least some dynamic component in most patients. The response to CRT might be modulated by the severity of IMR and the extent of LV remodeling before implantation. Severe IMR (ERO >20 mm2) in the setting of an enlarged LV is associated with lack of reverse remodeling during follow-up.

Coapsys Mitral Annuloplasty (Myocor)

The Coapsys device significantly reduced MR by significantly reducing the septal–lateral dimensions chronically at mitral annular level as well as at mid-papillary levels. This device has the advantage of being placed on a beating heart without CPB, and can be adjusted under echo guidance. It eliminates MR by decreasing annular dilatation as well as the papillary muscle displacement [52, 53]. Performing this technique off pump can help avoiding the possible complications associated with the use of CPB. Furthermore, immediate evaluation is possible as the device is being sized. The outcome of the annuloplasty ring placement cannot be adequately assessed until the patient is weaned from CPB. The complications associated with an inadequate repair result in added procedural and anesthetic times, and are among the reasons for increased morbidity/mortality rates in annuloplasty-treated patients.

RESULTS

Results of Mitral Valve Repair in Ischemic Mitral Regurgitation vs. Degenerative Mitral Regurgitation

MV repair has a survival advantage over MVR in patients with organic MR [54]. However, for IMR there is no clear benefit from MVr over MVR and further more, the outcome of patients with ischemic MR is more related to the patient's clinical status rather than to the type of procedure. This lack of clear benefits for MVr in IMR is related to the high risk of persistent MR after repair in IMR patients which is estimated to be 10% to 20% in addition to 50% to 70% rates of recurrent MR at 5 years [55]. The presence of persistent or recurrent MR is associated with higher incidence of cardiac events and reduced survival [56].

Revascularization Alone vs. Revascularization and Mitral Valve Repair for Ischemic Mitral Regurgitation

The striking, well-documented association of IMR and late survival has resulted in the hypothesis that eliminating severe MR at revascularization improves outcomes [16]. Additionally, the presence of moderate MR following CABG is associated with poor survival [57]. However, concomitant MV procedure has been consistently associated with significant increase in operative risk requiring prolonged surgical time, and the supposed benefit on long-term survival still needs to be demonstrated even in patients with severe MR [31, 32, 58-60]. Optimal treatment of significant IMR remains controversial. The explanation for the heterogeneous outcomes in IMR may be related to the fact that IMR is only a manifestation of advanced ventricular remodeling and that survival of these patients is primarily dictated by the extent of their ischemic heart disease. Available studies comparing CABG alone with CABG and MVr have been criticized for their small sample size, retrospective design, heterogeneity and selection bias related with the high-risk condition of this population. Meta-analysis of the pooled study population [61] showed that the addition of MV surgery did not have advantages on late mortality compared with CABG alone. Combined MV surgery was significantly associated with a lower residual MR grade compared with CABG alone. However, there was no effect on postoperative NYHA functional class or long-term survival.

Mitral Valve Repair vs. Replacement for Ischemic Mitral Regurgitation.

Restrictive mitral valve annuloplasty is currently the most frequently used technique for the surgical management of patients with severe IMR. However, IMR is in essence a ventricular and not a valvular disease and restrictive mitral annuloplasty targets the consequence rather than the cause of the disease. Consequently, this procedure was associated with 10% to 20% rates of persistent MR early after operation and with 50% to 70% rates of recurrent MR at 5 years [55]. Furthermore, the presence of persistent or recurrent MR is associated with higher incidence of cardiac events and reduced survival [56]. On the other hand, the outcome of patients undergoing MVR is influenced with the thromboembolic complications, which are important cause of morbidity and mortality in patients with a prosthetic valve. The risk of thromboembolic events is higher with mechanical than with bioprosthetic valves, and in the early versus late postoperative phases. Moreover, the rate of structural valve deterioration in bioprosthetic valves increases over time, particularly after the initial 8 to 10 years after implantation, and thereby exposes the patient to the risk of reoperation. Some studies reported that unadjusted survival is lower with MVR than with MVr in patients with ischemic MR [62, 63]. However, patients undergoing MVR are frequently older, sicker, and have more comorbidities than those with MVr, which may explain survival differences between the 2 treatment groups. Cohn et al [64] demonstrated that the outcome of patients with IMR is more related to the patient's clinical status rather than to the type of procedure (MVR versus MVr). Consistently, Grossi et al [65] reported that the type of procedure has little influence on prognosis after adjustment for preoperative NYHA class. Moreover, in their study, MVR provided better and more durable correction of

MR in the subset of patients with severe ventricular-papillary dysfunction. Lancelloti [66] repoted some predictors of poor outcomes after surgical treatment of IMR (table 1). Using propensity score-matched cohorts, Gillinov et al [67] found that MVr provides better postoperative outcomes compared to MVR. However, in high-risk patients, survival was similar with both types of procedure.

Several studies have demonstrated that it is possible to predict the risk of persistent MR and, to a lesser extent, the risk of recurrent MR after MVr from the preoperative echocardiographic evaluation [66] (Table 2). MVR or alternative procedures targeting the mitral valve apparatus or the LV should be contemplated in the patients identified as being at high risk for MVr failure based on preoperative echocardiography.

Future Prospective

Percutaneous Techniques

Several percutaneous modalities are currently investigated. Percutaneous edge-to-edge procedure (figure 5) has been proposed to reduce organic and also IMR, through the apposition of the centre of the two mitral leaflets, producing a double orifice [68]. Several interventions take advantage of the close proximity of the posterior mitral annulus to the coronary sinus.

Table 1. predictors of poor outcome after surgical treatment of IMR.

History	Condition	Echocardiography	Surgery
Older age Diabetes Mellitus Congestive heart Failure Advanced NYHA class Renal failure Associated comorbid conditions	High Euroscore Emergency operation Cardiogenic shock	LV EF < 30% Lack of viability and/ or myocardial scarring Severe LV remodeling Severe MV deformation Complex regurgitant jet Restrictive diastolic filling	left main stenosis Triple vessel disease MVR (vs. MVr) Residual MR (> +1)

Table 2. Echocardiographic predictors of MV repair failure:

Echo parameters	Threshold
Coaptation distance	≥ 1 cm
Systolic tenting area	> 2.5 cm^2
Posterolateral angle	> 45 °
Lateral wall motion abnormality	Scar
Central regurgitant jet	Absence
Complex regurgitant jets	Multiple
LVESD	≥ 51 mm
LVEDD	≥ 65 mm

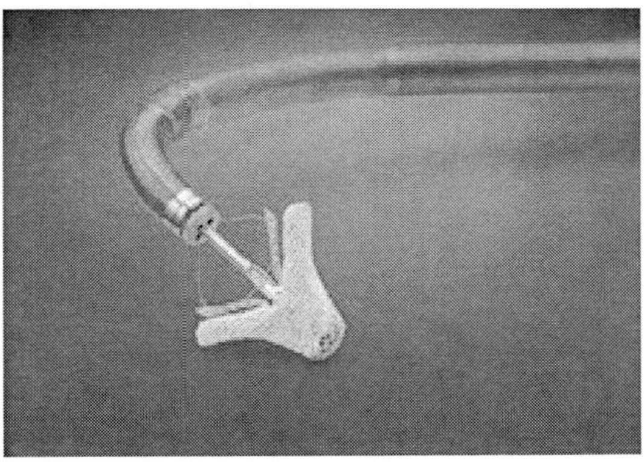

Figure 5. Mitral E Clip.

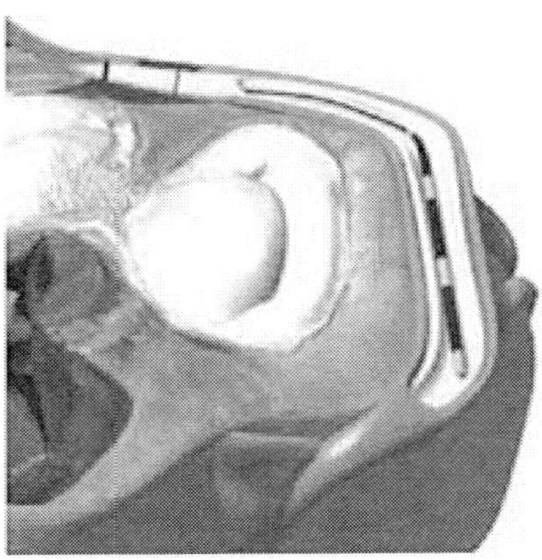

Figure 6. Percutaneous mitral valve annuloplasty through the coronary sinus.

These devices can be inserted into the coronary sinus to remodel the posterior portion of the annulus (figure 6), modify its shape and push the posterior leaflet forward, restoring mitral competence or at least, reducing the severity of MR [69, 70]. Although most devices can be inserted successfully and can reduce MR in the short term, maintenance of these effects over time and long-term clinical benefit remains to be established.

Future Therapeutic Targets

Autologous myoblast transplantation in the infarcted area has been used in an experimental model, showing the potential of decreasing IMR by a localized LV reverse remodeling [71]. The recently observed mitral leaflet adaptation to LV remodeling could potentially be in the future a therapeutic target when the mechanisms that underlie leaflet adaptation will be completely understood and if they can be potentially modified.

References

[1] Birnbaum Y, Chamoun AJ, Conti VR, et al: Mitral regurgitation following acute myocardial infarction. *Coron Artery Dis* 13:337-344, 2002.

[2] Levine RA, Schwammenthal E. Ischemic mitral regurgitation on the threshold of a solution: from paradoxes to unifying concepts. *Circulation* 2005;112:745–758.

[3] Borger MA, Alam A, Murphy PM, Doenst T, David TE. Chronic ischemic mitral regurgitation: repair, replace or rethink? *Ann Thorac Surg*. 2006;81:1153–1161.

[4] Bursi F, Enriquez-Sarano M, Jacobsen SJ, et al. Mitral regurgitation after myocardial infarction: a review. *Am J Med* 2006;119:103–12.

[5] Bursi F, Enriquez-Sarano M, Vuyisile T, et al. Heart failure and death after myocardial infarction in the community. The emerging role of mitral regurgitation. *Circulation* 2005;111:295–301.

[6] Tenenbaum A, Leor J, Motro M, et al. Improved posterobasal segment function after thrombolysis is associated with decreased incidence of significant mitral regurgitation in a first inferior myocardial infarction. *J Am Coll Cardiol* 1995;25:1558.

[7] Picard MH, Davidoff R, Sleeper LA, et al; SHOCK Trial. SHould we emergently revascularize Occluded Coronaries for cardiogenic shock. Echocardiographic predictors of survival and response to early revascularization in cardiogenic shock. *Circulation* 2003;107:279–84.

[8] Lancellotti P, Troisfontaines P, Toussaint A-C, et al. Prognostic importance of exercise-induced changes in mitral regurgitation in patients with chronic ischemic left ventricular dysfunction. *Circulation* 2003;108:1713–17.

[9] Schwammenthal E, Levine RA: The non-ischemic dynamics of ischemic mitral regurgitation: Solving the paradox. *Eur Heart* J 26:1454-1455, 2005.

[10] Yoran C, Yellin EL, Becker RM, et al: Dynamic aspects of acute mitral regurgitation: Effects of ventricular volume, pressure and contractility on the effective regurgitant orifice area. *Circulation* 60:170-176, 1979.

[11] Schwammenthal E, Chen C, Benning F, et al: Dynamics of mitral regurgitant flow and orifice area. Physiologic application of the proximal flow convergence method: Clinical data and experimental testing. *Circulation* 90:307-322, 1994.

[12] He S, Fontaine AA, Schwammenthal E, et al: Integrated mechanism for functional mitral regurgitation: Leaflet restriction versus coapting force: In vitro studies. *Circulation* 96:1826-1834, 1997.

[13] Lehmann KG, Francis CK, Dodge HT, the TIMI Study Group. Mitral regurgitation in the early myocardial infarction. *Ann Intern Med* 1992;117:10–17.

[14] Bursi F, Enriquez-Sarano M, Nkomo VT, Jacobsen ST, Westo SA, Meverden RA, Roger VL. Heart failure and death after myocardial infarction in the community: the emerging role of mitral regurgitation. *Circulation* 2005;111:295–301.

[15] Grigioni F, Enriquez-Sarano M, Zehr KJ, Bailey KR, Tajik AJ. Ischemic mitral regurgitation: long-term outcome and prognostic implications with quantitative Doppler assessment. *Circulation* 2001;103:1759–1764.

[16] Aronson D, Goldsher N, Zukermann R, et al.: Ischemic mitral regurgitation and risk of heart failure after myocardial infarction. *Arch Intern Med* 2006, 166:2362–2368.

[17] Lancellotti P, Ge´rard PL, Pie´rard LA. Long-term outcome of patients with heart failure and dynamic functional mitral regurgitation. *Eur Heart J* 2005;26: 1528–1532.

[18] Lancellotti P, Lebrun F, Pie´rard LA. Determinants of exercise-induced changes in mitral regurgitation in patients with coronary artery disease and left ventricular dysfunction. *J Am Coll Cardiol* 2003;42:1921–1928.

[19] Yosefy C, Levine RA, Solis J, Vaturi M, Handschumacher MD, Hung J. Proximal flow convergence region as assessed by real-time 3-dimensional echocardiography: challenging the hemispheric assumption. *J Am Soc Echocardiogr* 2007;20: 389–396.

[20] Ryan LP, Salgo IS, Gorman RC, Gorman JH 3rd: The emerging role of three-dimensional echocardiography in mitral valve repair. *Semin Thorac Cardiovasc Surg* 2006, 18:126–134.

[21] Ryan L, Jackson B, Parish L, et al.: Quantifi cation and localization of mitral valve tenting in ischemic mitral regurgitation using real-time three-dimensional echocardiography. *Eur J Cardiothorac Surg* 2007, 31:839–834.

[22] Lebrun F, Lancellotti P, Pie´rard LA. Quantitation of functional mitral regurgitation during bicycle exercise in patients with heart failure. *J Am Coll Cardiol* 2001;38: 1685–1692.

[23] Lancellotti P, Stainier PY, Lebois F, Pie´rard L. Effect of dynamic left ventricular dyssynchrony on dynamic mitral regurgitation in patients with heart failure due to coronary artery disease. *Am J Cardiol* 2005;96:1304–1307.

[24] Kuhl HP, Papavasiliu TS, Beek AM, Hofman MB, Heusen NS, van Rossum AC. Myocardial viability: rapid assessment with delayed contrast-enhanced MR imaging with three-dimensional inversion ecovery prepared pulse sequence. *Radiology*. 2004;230:576 –582.

[25] Penicka M, Linkova H, Lang O, Fojt R, Kocka V, Vanderheyden M, Bartunek J. Predictors of improvement of unrepaired moderate ischemic mitral regurgitation in patients undergoing elective isolated coronary artery bypass graft surgery. *Circulation.* 2009;120:1474 –1481.

[26] Tavakoli R, Weber A, Vogt P, Brunner HP, Pretre R, Turina M. Surgical management of acute mitral valve regurgitation due to post-infarction papillary muscle rupture. *J Heart Valve Dis* 2002; 11:20 –5.

[27] Tolis GA Jr., Korkolis DP, Kopf GS, Elefteriades JA. Revascularization alone (without mitral valve repair) suffices in patients with advanced ischemic cardiomyopathy and mild-to-moderate mitral regurgitation. *Ann Thorac Surg* 2002;74:1476–80.

[28] Lam BK, Gillinov AM, Blackstone EH, et al. Importance of moderate ischemic mitral regurgitation. *Ann Thorac Surg* 2005;79: 462–70.
[29] Schroder JN, Williams ML, Hata JA, et al. Impact of mitral valve regurgitation evaluated by intraoperative transesophageal echocardio graphy on long-term outcomes after coronary artery bypass grafting. *Circulation* 2005;112:I293– 8.
[30] Aklog L, Filsoufi F, Flores KQ, et al. Does coronary artery bypass grafting alone correct moderate ischemic mitral regurgitation? *Circulation* 2001;104:I68 –75.
[31] Harris KM, Sundt TM III, Aeppli D, Sharma R, Barzilai B. Can late survival of patients with moderate ischemic mitral regurgitation be impacted by intervention on the valve? *Ann Thorac Surg* 2002;74:1468 –75.
[32] Kang DH, Kim MJ, Kang SJ, et al. Mitral valve repair versus revascularization alone in the treatment of ischemic mitral regurgitation. *Circulation* 2006;114:I499–503.
[33] Lancellotti P, Donal E, Cosyns B, et al. Effects of surgery on ischaemic mitral regurgitation: a prospective multicenter registry (SIMRAM registry). *Eur J Echocardiogr* 2008;9:26–30.
[34] McGee EC, Gillinov MA, Blackstone EH, et al. Recurrent mitral regurgitation after annuloplasty for functional ischemic mitral regurgitation. *J Thorac Cardiovasc Surg*. 2004;128:916 –924.
[35] Hung J, Papakostas L, Tahta SA, et al. Mechanism of recurrent ischemic mitral regurgitation after annuloplasty. Continued LV remodeling as a moving target. *Circulation.* 2004;110 (suppl II):II-85–II-90.
[36] Braun J, van de Veire NR, Klautz RJ, et al.: Restrictive mitral annuloplasty cures ischemic mitral regurgitation and heart failure. *Ann Thorac Surg* 2008, 85:430–436.
[37] Daimon M, Fukuda S, Adams DH, et al. Mitral valve repair with Carpentier- McCarthy-Adams IMR ETlogix annuloplasty ring for ischemic mitral regurgitation: early echocardiographic results from a multi-center study. *Circulation.* 2006;114 (suppl I):I-588 –I-593.
[38] Langer F, Rodriguez S, Cheng A, Ortiz S, Nguyen TC, Zasio MK, Liang D, Daughters GT, Ingels NB, Miller DC. Posterior mitral leaflet extension: an adjunctive repair option for ischemic mitral regurgitation? *J Thorac Cardiovasc Surg.* 2006;131:868–877.

[39] De Varennes B, Chaturvedi R, Sidhu S, Côté AV, Shan WL, Goyer C, Hatzakorzian R, Buithieu J and Sniderman A. Initial Results of Posterior Leaflet Extension for Severe Type IIIb Ischemic Mitral Regurgitation. *Circulation* 2009; 119;2837-2843.

[40] Kincaid EH, Riley RD, Hines MH, et al. Anterior leaflet augmentation for ischemic mitral regurgitation. *Ann Thorac Surg*. 2004;78:564 –568.

[41] Hung J, Chaput M, Guerrero JL, et al.: Persistent reduction of ischemic mitral regurgitation by papillary muscle repositioning: structural stabilization of the papillary muscle-ventricular wall complex. *Circulation* 2007, 116 (11 Suppl):I259–I263.

[42] Kron IL, Green GR, Cope JT: Surgical relocation of the posterior papillary muscle in chronic ischemic mitral regurgitation. *Ann Thorac Surg* 2002, 74:600–601.

[43] Gazoni LM, Kern JA, Swenson BR, et al.: A change in perspective: results for ischemic mitral valve repair are similar to mitral valve repair for degenerative disease. *Ann Thorac Surg* 2007, 84:750–757.

[44] Ramadan R, Al-Attar N, Mohammadi S, et al. Left ventricular infarct plication restores mitral function in chronic ischemic mitral regurgitation. *J Thorac Cardiovasc Surg*. 2005;129:440–442.

[45] Borger MA, Murphy PM, Alam A, et al.: Initial results of the chordal-cutting operation for ischemic mitral regurgitation. *J Thorac Cardiovasc Surg* 2007, 133:1483–1492.

[46] Alfieri O, Maisano F, De Bonis M, et al. The double-orifice technique in mitral valve repair: a simple solution for complex problems. *J Thorac Cardiovasc Surg.* 2001;122:677– 681.

[47] Maisano F, Caldarola A, Blasio A, et al. Midterm results of edge-to-edge mitral valve repair without annuloplasty. *J Thorac Cardiovasc Surg*. 2003; 126:1987–1997.

[48] Gillinov AM: Is ischemic mitral regurgitation an indication for surgical repair or replacement? *Heart Fail Rev* 2006, 11:231–239.

[49] Kanzaki H, Bazaz R, Schwartzman D, et al. A mechanism for immediate reduction in mitral regurgitation after cardiac resynchronization therapy. *J Am Coll Cardiol* 2004;44:1619–25.

[50] Sutton MG, Plappert T, Hilpisch KE, et al. Sustained reverse left ventricular structural remodeling with cardiac resynchronization at one year is a function of etiology: quantitative Doppler echocardiographic evidence from the Multicenter InSync Randomized Clinical Evaluation (MIRACLE). *Circulation* 2006;113:266–72.

[51] Madaric J, Vanderheyden M, Van Laethem C, et al. Early and late effects of cardiac resynchronization therapy on exercise-induced mitral regurgitation: relationship with left ventricular dyssynchrony, re-modelling and cardiopulmonary performance. *Eur Heart J* 2007;28:2134–41.

[52] Tibayan FA, Rodriguez F, Zasio MK, Bailey L, Liang D, Daughters GT, Langer F, Ingels Jr. NB, Miller DC. Geometric distortions of the mitral valvular–ventricular complex in chronic ischemic mitral regurgitation. *Circulation* 2003;108 (Suppl 1):II116–21.

[53] Fukamachi K, Popovic ZB, Inoue M, Doi K, Schenk S, Ootaki Y, Kopcak MW, McCarthy PM. Changes in mitral annular and left ventricular dimensions and left ventricular pressure–volume relations after off-pump treatment of mitral regurgitation with the Coapsys device. *Eur J Cardiothorac Surg* 2004;25:352-357

[54] Enriquez-Sarano M, Schaff HV, Frye RL. Mitral regurgitation: what causes the leakage is fundamental to the outcome of valve repair. *Circulation*. 2003; 108:253–256.

[55] Magne J, Se´ne´chal M, Dumesnil JG, Pibarot P. Ischemic mitral regurgitation: a complex multifaceted disease. *Cardiology*. 2009; 112:244–259.

[56] Serri K, Bouchard D, Demers P, Coutu M, Pellerin M, Carrier M, Perrault LP, Cartier R, Page P, Cossette M, Basmadjian AJ. Is a good perioperative echocardiographic result predictive of durability in ischemic mitral valve repair? *J Thorac Cardiovasc Surg*. 2006; 131:565–573.

[57] Crabtree TD, Bailey MS, Moon MR, Munfakh N, Pasque MK, Lawton JS, et al. Recurrent mitral regurgitation and risk factors for early and late mortality after mitral valve repair for functional ischemic mitral regurgitation. *Ann Thorac Surg* 2008; 85:1537–1542.

[58] Diodato MD, Moon MR, Pasque MK, Barner HB, Moazami N, Lawton JS, et al. Repair of ischemic mitral regurgitation does not increase mortality or improve long-term survival in patients undergoing coronary artery revascularization: a propensity analysis. *Ann Thorac Surg* 2004; 78:794–799.

[59] Mihaljevic T, Lam BK, Rajeswaran J, Takagaki M, Lauer MS, Gillinov AM, et al. Impact of mitral valve annuloplasty combined with revascularization in patients with functional ischemic mitral regurgitation. *J Am Coll Cardiol* 2007; 49:2191–2201.

[60] Prifti E, Bonacchi M, Frati G, Giunti G, Babatasi G, Sani G. Ischemic mitral valve regurgitation grade II-III: correction in patients with impaired left ventricular function undergoing simultaneous coronary revascularization. *J Heart Valve Dis* 2001; 10:754–762.

[61] Benedetto U, Melina G, Roscitano A, Fiorani B, Capuano F, Sclafani G, Comito C, di Nucci GD and Sinatra R. Does combined mitral valve surgery improve survival when compared to revascularization alone in patients with ischemic mitral regurgitation? A meta-analysis on 2479 patients. *Journal of Cardiovascular Medicine* 2009, 10:109–114.

[62] Al-Radi OO, Austin PC, Tu JV, David TE, Yau TM. Mitral repair versus replacement for ischemic mitral regurgitation. *Ann Thorac Surg.* 2005; 79:1260 –1267.

[63] Thourani VH, Weintraub WS, Guyton RA, Jones EL, Williams WH, Elkabbani S, Craver JM. Outcomes and long-term survival for patients Undergoing mitral valve repair versus replacement. Effect of age and concomitant artery bypass grafting. *Circulation.* 2003;108:298 –304.

[64] Cohn L.H, Rizzo RJ, Adams DH, Couper GS, Sullivan TE, Collins JJ. The effect of pathophysiology on the surgical treatment of ischemic mitral regurgitation: operative and late risks of repair versus replacement. *Eur J Cardiothorac Surg.* 1995;9:568 –574.

[65] Grossi EA, Goldberg JD, LaPietra A, Ye X, Zakow P, Sussman M, Delianides J, Culliford AT, Esposito RA, Ribakove GH, Galloway AC, Colvin SB. Ischemic mitral valve reconstruction and replacement: comparison of long-term survival and complications. *J Thorac Cardiovasc Surg*. 2001;122:1107–1124.

[66] Lancellotti P, Marwick T, Pierard LA. How to manage ischaemic mitral Regurgitation. *Heart* 2008;94:1497–1502

[67] Gillinov AM, Wierup PN, Blackstone EH, Bishay ES, Cosgrove DM, White J, Lytle BW, McCarthy PM. Is repair preferable to replacement for ischemic mitral regurgitation? *J Thorac Cardiovasc Surg*. 2001;122: 1125–1141.

[68] De Bonis M, Lapenna E, La Canna G, Ficarra E, Pagliaro M, Torracca L, Maisano F, Alfieri O. Mitral valve repair for functional mitral regurgitation in end-stage dilated cardiomyopathy: role of the 'edge-to-edge' technique. *Circulation* 2005;112: I402–I408.

[69] Webb JG, Hamek J, Munt BI, Kimblad PO, Chandavimol M, Thompson CR, Mayo JR, Solem JO. Percutaneous transvenous mitral annuloplasty. Initial human experience with device implantation in the coronary sinus. *Circulation* 2006;113: 851–855.

[70] Sack S, Kahlert P, Bilodeau L, Pie´rard LA, Lancellotti P, Legrand V, Bartunek J, Vanderheyden M, Hoffmann R, Schauerte P, Shiota T, Marks DS, Erbel R, Ellis SG. Percutaneous transvenous mitral annuloplasty: initial human experience with a novel coronary sinus implant device. *Circ Cardiovasc Interv* 2009;2:277–284.

[71] Messas E, Bel A, Morichetti M, Carrion C, Handschumacher MD, Peyrard S, Vilquin JT, Desnos M, Bruneval P, Carpentier A, Menasche´ P, Levine RA, Hage`ge AA. Autologous myoblast transplantation for chronic ischemic mitral regurgitation. *J Am Coll Cardiol* 2006;47:2086–2093.

In: Mitral Valve Disease
Editor: Richard R. Heuser
ISBN: 978-1-61942-309-1

Chapter 3

INFECTIVE ENDOCARDITIS OF THE MITRAL VALVE

Tadashi Omoto, Takeo Tedoriya, Tadamasa Miyauchi and Noboru Ishikawa
Division of Thoracic and Cardiovascular Surgery, Department of Surgery, Showa University, School of Medicine, Tokyo, Japan

INTRODUCTION

Surgical strategies for the treatment of infective endocarditis (IE) of the mitral valve (MV) remain controversial. MV repair has recently assumed popularity over MV replacement due to its benefits in preserving ventricular function and avoiding the use of a prosthetic valve [1-3] particularly during the active-stage with continued fever, septicemia, septic emboli, or acute heart failure. This chapter outlines current thinking in surgical intervention for MV during active-stage IE.

ACTIVE-STAGE IE

Assessment of patients with IE requires an accurate appreciation of disease process stage. Definitions of active IE vary: Doukas and colleagues diagnose active disease when a positive blood culture is obtained in the three weeks before surgery or when culture of the excised valve is positive [4]; Manhas and colleagues when hemodynamic deterioration or the presence of large (>10mm) vegetations or systemic emboli lead to surgery [5]; and Dreyfus and colleagues when surgery is performed during the first 6 weeks of antibiotic therapy [6]. Allowing for these variations, IE generally considered active when an operation is required before a standard course of antibiotic treatment is completed.

The question of whether MV surgery should be done during the active or healed stage depends on the virulence of the causative microorganism (drug-resistant organism, *Staphylococcus aureus*, or fungus), embolic events, effectiveness of antibiotic therapy and immunological aspects. Despite ongoing refinement of surgical and antibiotic therapies, early mortality for patients with active-stage IE remains high. In their study of 71 consecutive patients who underwent MV surgery for IE, Lee and colleagues [7] found that 30-day mortality was low in healed IE (3.3%) but quite high (29%) in the active phase. High mortality in active-stage IE is associated with causative microorganism (higher mortality in cases due to *Staphylococcus aureus* [7]), poor ventricular function [8,9] and poor preoperative condition. David and colleagues reviewed 266 patients with active-stage IE who underwent surgery for MV and showed that patients with impaired LV function (EF<40%) had high operative mortality compared with overall mortality (14% vs. 9%) [2]. Ruttman and colleagues reviewed 68 patients with active-stage IE who underwent MV operation and showed that impaired LV function (EF<48%) was associated with poor event-free survival at 5 years [3]. These studies indicate that early mortality might be improved if the patient undergoes earlier operation before ventricular performance has changed from the compensated state (LV dilatation with increased LV end-systolic dimension) to the decompensated state (LV dilatation without increased LV end-systolic dimension). Further, they also indicate that early mortality in active-stage IE may be improved by MV repair, thanks to its preservation of LV function via its preservation of leaflet-papillary muscle-LV continuity.

The preoperative condition of patients requiring surgery while infection is still uncontrolled is unsurprisingly poor, particularly those with "hospital-acquired endocarditis" as a result of methicillin-resistant Staphylococcus aureus (MRSA) or methicillin-resistant coagulase-negative staphylococci (MRCNS). Hospital-acquired endocarditis has been defined as IE with an onset greater than 72 hours after admission or IE acquired in association with a significant invasive procedure performed during hospitalization less than 8 weeks before onset [8,9]. Hospital-acquired endocarditis is characteristically associated with hemodialysis, dependence on intravenous nutritional support, chemotherapy for malignancy, or respirator use, and is characterized by a bacterial spectrum which is distinct from that of community-acquired IE. MRSA, MRCNS, and enteric gram negative bacilli are strongly associated with hospital-acquired endocarditis [10,11]. Postoperative prognosis is poor, with mortality rates of around 50% [8,9], likely attributable to the immuno-compromised state of these patients. If the preoperative condition is evaluated as severely comorbid, antibiotic therapy will be less effective than expected and MV surgery should be undertaken on an emergency basis, because destruction of the leaflets and subvalvular apparatus will progress by the hour. The benefits of MV repair may be more strongly apparent in patients with hospital-acquired endocarditis because of their lower nutritional state, which may involve a higher risk of postoperative re-infection; and poor circulatory status, which may confer a higher risk of postoperative low output syndrome

PRINCIPLES OF SURGICAL INDICATION

Indications for surgery are based on the specific disease course, degree of tissue destruction, hemodynamics and complications in the individual patient. Any comorbid conditions must also be taken into account.

In principle, surgical intervention is recommended in three clinical situations:

1. Persistent infection that is unresponsive to appropriate antibiotic therapy. If fever pattern, leukocytosis, or CRP do not change, the patient is assessed as unresponsive to medical therapy. In these cases, the echocardiogram usually shows large vegetation and subvalvular extension.
2. Progressive heart failure–this usually requires early surgical intervention because it indicates that valvular destruction has reached the threshold at which acute valvular regurgitation progresses to the decompensated state. The echocardiogram shows left ventricular (LV) dilatation with an increase in LV end-systolic dimension as well as LV end-diastolic dimension. LV ejection fraction (EF) decreases and the severity of secondary tricuspid regurgitation worsens.

3. Recurrent embolic events - early surgical intervention prevents fatal complications resulting from further embolization, such as hemorrhagic cerebral infarction. The echocardiogram shows vegetation which is large, fragile and mobile.

The echocardiogram may show small vegetations (3-5mm) with moderate mitral regurgitation (MR) and preserved LV function. Serial echocardiograms are important in following up changes in vegetation size, subvalvular extension, and degree of MR and LV performance. A small increase in LV volume overload may be reflected by an increase in transvalvular peak gradient of the tricuspid valve without changes in LV structure or mitral regurgitant volume. Intracardiac infective foci may progress in patients with comorbidities or IE caused by virulent organisms, and early surgery may be warranted.

Neurological Complications

The rate of neurological complications in patients with IE is high, ranging from 25%-40% in those with left heart endocarditis [12-14], and occurring more frequently in MV IE than aortic valve IE [15]. Anderson and colleagues reviewed 707 patients with definite or possible IE and demonstrated that those with MV IE had a 1.8 times higher risk of stroke than those with aortic valve IE [15]. The spectrum of neurologic events includes cerebral infarction, hemorrhagic cerebral infarction, mycotic aneurysm, meningitis, and brain abscess [12-15]. Neurological complications associated with cardiac surgery include: (1) anticoagulation therapy with heparin may exacerbate hemorrhagic infarction and convert non-hemorrhagic to hemorrhagic cerebral infarction, (2) hypotension during CPB may aggravate preexisting ischemic neurologic injury, and (3) CPB may potentiate cerebral edema in areas of blood-brain barrier disruption [16]. The establishment of guidelines for patient evaluation and the timing of surgery are hampered by the limited surgical experience in single institutions, and the small sample size of most clinical studies. One of the largest series examining valve replacement in patients with cerebral infarction was reported by Ting and colleagues from the University of Illinois [17]: in their study, mean interval from the onset of neurologic deficit to cardiac operation was 11.4 days; no patient with non-hemorrhagic cerebral infarction sustained a perioperative stroke; only preoperative hemorrhage on CT scan correlated with mortality and perioperative stroke; and the timing of operation was not related with outcome. Previous studies of timing strategies recommended a delay of 2 to 3 weeks for patients with non-hemorrhagic cerebral infarction [18]. Although few studies have investigated timing in patients with active IE who experience intracranial hemorrhage, an interval of 4 weeks between the neurologic event and cardiac operation is warranted in stable patients [18]. If a ruptured mycotic aneurysm is present, this must be resected, clipped or embolized before cardiac surgery [19].

Principles of Surgery

The two key principles of MV repair in active-stage IE are aggressive debridement of infected tissue and leaflet repair using tissue which ensures the security and long-term durability of the suture. The preoperative echocardiogram is important in establishing the surgical strategy and will divide IE in the MV into two categories, the *central type* and the *commissural type*. Patients categorized into both types will experience massive MV insufficiency and severe heart failure. The *central type* is often repaired by partial leaflet resection of the anterior mitral leaflet (AML) and leaflet resection of the posterior mitral leaflet (PML). MV repair with resection of less than 1/3 of the leaflet is highly feasible, even if the vegetation is large. Large resection of the AML with multiple artificial chordae may result in coaptation failure, but smaller resection of the AML can be reconstructed by autologous pericardial patching. After leaflet resection of the P2 scallop the PML can be reconstructed by the leaflet sliding technique and annular compression sutures. We prefer to use a prosthetic annular ring to ensure good coaptation of leaflets and a reduction in suture tension [1]. Infection of the annular ring after MV repair appears rare. The *commissural type* is often associated with bileaflet resection and requires patch repair using glutaraldehyde autologous pericardium. Large vegetation on echocardiography may be a complex of infective tissue and torn chordae, and MV repair may require the implantation of multiple artificial chordae. If vegetation is also demonstrated in the aortic valve, the infective lesion in the MV is often very severe: the feasibility of MV repair is in these cases is low, and they should rather be treated by substantial leaflet and subvalvular tissue excision.

Significances of MV Repair in Patients with Active-stage IE

The role of MV repair in the management of active-stage IE is an important issue in studies of native IE. MV repair with large leaflet defects may results in residual MR in the long-term, but better LV function and the avoidance of warfarin therapy are major benefits in the preoperative management of high-risk patients. Omoto and colleagues reviewed 22 consecutive operations for native MV active IE at Showa University Hospital [20]. MV repair was performed in 15 patients (68.2%), of whom 3 required re-operation. Two of three patients had progression of MR despite a finding by intraoperative transesophageal echocardiography that the MR was less than mild. Recurrence of MR was associated with the durability of MV repair, with dehiscence of the patch in both patients, and repeat MV repair being feasible in one. One patient with mild to moderate MR sustained hemolysis, which might have been due to either or both the prosthetic ring or artificial chordae, or to high shear stress caused by the regurgitant flow after repair. Testing of hemodynamics, ventricular function and ventricular structure showed that the recurrence of MR was well-tolerated in all three patients, and the tissue was less friable and held sutures better in the healed stage of IE. Furthermore, repeat surgery after MV repair has an advantage in the strength of the preserved mitral annulus, which results in less long-term risk of paravalvular leakage.

In many patients, greater severity of infection is associated with a lower feasibility of MV repair; in particular, aortic valve involvement, recurrent embolic episodes, and the comorbidities associated with them increases postoperative bleeding complications, including intracranial and gastrointestinal bleeding. In these cases, the better early mortality and morbidities with bio-prosthesis make it generally preferable, even though it may also require re-operation for structural valve deterioration in the long-term.

Given the relatively high mortality with MV surgery in patients with active-stage IE, greater emphasis should be placed on the early mortality advantage provided by MV repair. The feasibility of MV repair in patients with degenerative MV disease is important, because residual MR may require future re-operation. The goal of MV repair in patients with active-stage IE is to reduce early mortality by controlling infection and improving LV function and structure. Greater use of MV repair in patients with active-stage IE would increase the occurrence of postoperative residual MR, but would be justified if it improved early mortality.

An additional risk in patients who undergo MV replacement during active-stage IE is the recurrence of infection. Rutmann and colleagues reported that actuarial freedom from recurrence of endocarditis at 5 years' follow-up was 96.4% after MV repair and 82.7% after MV replacement [3]. Fedoruk and colleagues reviewed 358 patients with active-stage IE who underwent MV replacement and reported that freedom from recurrent prosthetic valve endocarditis was 78.9% at 15 years [21]. Despite prompt diagnosis and the frequent use of surgical intervention, prosthetic valve endocarditis carries a worse outcome than native IE [2,22]. MV repair in active-phase IE is associated with lower rates of recurrence of infection than MV replacement and contributes to a better long-term outcome.

MVP in patients with active-stage IE is associated with a better ejection fraction and greater regression in ventricular dimension than valve replacement in the early postoperative period. Particular care should be taken in cases with a large patch repair after extensive leaflet resection, which may have less durability and a higher risk of recurrence of MR.

CONCLUSION

MV repair is preferable to MV replacement because it offers fewer thromboembolic complications, a lower risk of recurrence of endocarditis and better ventricular function. Early surgical intervention of IE prevents the progression of valvular destruction and embolic events. Nevertheless, while the feasibility of MV repair in the healed stage of IE is reasonably high, repair in active-stage IE sometimes requires complicated valve procedures involving multiple artificial chordae and large patch reconstruction, which in the long term are associated with residual MR or re-operation. The feasibility of MV repair should be carefully discussed with reference to the location of infective foci, valvular or subvalvular destruction, and the quality and quantity of valvular regurgitation.

REFERENCES

[1] Omoto T, Ohno M, Fukuzumi M, Ohi M, Okayama T, Ishikawa N, Tedoriya T. Mitral valve repair for infective endocarditis. *Gen Thorac Cardiovasc Surg* 2008;56:277-280.

[2] David TE, Gavra G, Feindel CM, Regesta T, Armstrong S, Maganti MD. Surgical treatment of active infective endocarditis: a continued challenge. *J Thorac Cardiovasc Surg* 2007;133:1444-149.

[3] Ruttman E, Legit C, Poelzl G, Mueller S, Chevtchik O, Cottogni M, Ulmer H, Pachinger O, Laufer G, Mueller LC. Mitral valve repair provides improved outcome over replacement in active infective endocarditis. *J Thorac Cardiovasc Surg* 2005;130:765-771.

[4] Doukas G, Oc M, Alexiou C, et al. Mitral valve repair for active culture positive infective endocarditis. *Heart* 2006;92:261-3.

[5] Manhas DR, Mohri H, Hessel EA, Merendino KA. Experience with surgical management of primary infective endocarditis: a collected review of 139 patients. *Am Heart J* 1972;84:738-47.

[6] Dreyfus G, Serraf A, Jebara VA, Deloche A, Chauvaud S, Couetil JP, et al. Valve repair in acute endocarditis. Ann Thorac Surg 1990;49:706-13.

[7] Lee EM, Shapiro LM, Wells FC. Conservative operation for infective endocarditis of the mitral valve. *Ann Thorac Surg* 1998;65:1087-92.

[8] Terpenning MS, Buggy BP, Kauffman CA. Hospital-acquired infective endocarditis. *Arch Intern Med* 1988;148:1601-3.

[9] Chen SC, Dwyer DE. Sorrell TC. A comparison of hospital and community-acquired infective endocarditis. *Am J Cardiol* 1992;70:1449-52.

[10] Jarvis WR, Martone WJ. Predominant pathogens in hospital infections. *J Antimicrob Chemother* 1992;29 (Suppl A):19-24.

[11] Sheikh AM, Elhenawy AM, Maganti M, Armstrong S, David TE, Feindel CM. Outcomes of double valve surgery for active infective endocarditis. *J Thorac Cardiovasc Surg* 2009;138:69-75.

[12] Heiro M, Nikoskelainen J, Endblom E, Kotilainen E, Marttila R, Kotilainen P. Neurologic manifestations of infective endocarditis: a 17-year experience in a teaching hospital in Finland. *Arch Intern Med* 2000;160:2781-2787.

[13] Hart RG, Foster JW, Luther MF, Kanter MC. Stroke in infective endocarditis. *Stroke* 1990;21:695-700.

[14] Ting W, Silverman N, Levitsky S. Valve replacement in patients with endocarditis and cerebral septic emboli. *Ann Thorac Surg* 1991;51:18-22.

[15] Anderson DJ, Goldstein LB, Wilkinson WE, Corey GR, Cabell CH, Sanders LL, Sexton DJ. Stroke location, characterization, severity, and outcome in mitral vs aortic valve endcarditis. *Neurology* 2003;61:1341-46.

[16] Zisbrod Z, Rose DM, Jacobowitz IJ, Kramer M, Acinapura AJ, Cunningham JN. Results of open heart surgery in patients with recent cardiogenic embolic stroke and central nervous system dysfunction. *Circulation* 1987;76 (suppl 5):109-12.

[17] Ting W, Silverman N, Levitsky S. Valve replacement in patients with endocarditis and cerebral septic emboli. *Ann Thorac Surg* 1991;51:18-22.

[18] Gillinov AM, Shah RV, Curtis W, Stuart RS, Cameron DE, Baumgartner WA, Greene PS. Valve replacement in patients with endocarditis and acute neurologic deficit. *Ann Thorac Surg* 1996;61:1125-30.

[19] D'Udekem Y, David TE, Feindel CM, et al. Long-term results of surgery for active infective endocarditis. *Eur J Cardiothorac Surg* 1997;11:46-52.

[20] Omoto T, Tedoriya T, Oi M, Nagano N, Miyauchi T, Ishikawa N. Significance of mitral valve repair for active-phase infective endocarditis. *Asian Ann Cardiovasc Thorac Ann* 2011;19:149-153.

[21] Fedoruk LM, Jamieson WR, Ling H, MacNab JS, Germann E, Karim SS, et al. Predictors of recurrence and reoperation for prosthetic valve endocarditis after valve replacement surgery for native valve endocarditis. *J Thorac Cardiovasc Surg* 2009;137:326-333.

[22] Wang A, Athan E, Pappas PA, Fowler JrVG, Olaison L, Pare C, et al. Contemporary clinical profile and outcome of prosthetic valve endocarditis. *JAMA* 2007;28:1354-1361.

.

In: Mitral Valve Disease
Editor: Richard R. Heuser
ISBN: 978-1-61942-309-1

Chapter 4

ASSESSMENT OF MITRAL VALVE DISEASE USING TWO DIMENSIONAL AND THREE- DIMENSIONAL ECHOCARDIOGRAPHY

***Hanan B. Albacker*[1], *Andrej Alfirevic*[2], *and Turki B. Albacker*[3]**

[1]Director of Non-Invasive & Echocardiography Laboratories Department of Cardiology, King Fahad Cardiac Center, King Khalid Medical City, King Saud University, Riyadh, Saudi Arabia
[2]Director of perioperative Echocardiography, Department of Thoracic & Cardiovascular Anesthesia, Heart & Vascular Institute, Cleveland Clinic Foundation, Cleveland, US
[3]Department of Cardiac Surgery, King Fahad Cardiac Center, King Khalid Medical City, King Saud University, Riyadh, Saudi Arabia

ABSTRACT

Mitral valve disease is a common disease that requires an accurate evaluation of mitral valve structural changes and their hemodynamic significance. In cases of mitral valve regurgitation, Evaluation of disease severity and its effect on myocardial function plays an important role on choosing the appropriate treatment modality and its timing. When surgical treatment is indicated, pre-operative assessment of MV anatomy is essential for surgical planning and design in patients undergoing MV repair. Although two-dimensional (2D) echocardiography provides precise information regarding MV anatomy, three-dimensional (3D) echocardiography could increase the understanding of MV apparatus and individual scallop identification. Real time 3D (RT3D) transesophageal echocardiogram allows accurate and feasible identification of prolapse or flail of individual segments of MV leaflets during surgery. Echo cardiography is also an important tool for management of patients with mitral valve stenosis. To define the best therapeutic strategy in patients with mitral valve stenosis, clinical data and accurate measurements of mitral valve area (MVA) are necessary. Doppler-based methods are heavily influenced by hemodynamic variables, and associated valvular disease. Direct measurements of the MVA could traditionally only be performed using a planimetry traced on 2D echo images. However, this method has multiple limitations; the major one being the correct image plane orientation. RT-3D echocardiography provides a unique 'en-face' view of the complete mitral valve apparatus and has been shown to improve the accuracy of 2D echo MVA planimetry. RT3D echo provides a similari nter-observer variability compared with the pressure half-time method and shows a better inter-observer agreement than 2D echo for the assessment of the pre-valvuloplasty Wilkins score. 2D and 3D echocardio graphy should be regarded as complementary, not competitive, imaging modalities in patients with complex MV anatomy. Formal 3D echocardio graphic training should be encouraged and its use should be expanded use of in routine clinical practice. We review in this chapter the clinical uses of 2D and 3D echocardiography in assessment of mitral valve disease including up to date literature on this subject.

INTRODUCTION

Mitral valve disease is a common disease that requires an accurate evaluation of mitral valve structural changes and their hemodynamic significance. Evaluation of disease severity and its effect on myocardial function plays an important role on choosing the appropriate treatment modality and its timing. When surgical treatment is indicated, pre-operative assessment of mitral valve (MV) anatomy is essential for surgical planning as well as determining valve repairability and type of repair. Although two-dimensional (2D) echocardiography provides precise information regarding MV anatomy, three-dimensional (3D) echocardiography could increase the understanding of MV apparatus and individual scallop identification [1]. 2D and 3D echocardiography should be regarded as complementary, not competitive, imaging modalities in patients with complex MV anatomy. Functionally, the MV apparatus consists of several components: left atrial (LA) wall, mitral annulus, anterior and posterior leaflets, chordae and papillary muscles. Valvular regurgitation may be due to congenital or acquired abnormalities of the valve leaflets or to abnormalities of the associated supporting structures. For example, left ventricular (LV) dilation can result in mitral regurgitation (MR) even with normal valve leaflets and chordae. Echocardiographic examinations allow definition of the etiology of valvular regurgitation in most cases. Even when a single definite etiology is not evident, the differential diagnosis of the cause of regurgitation often can be narrowed to the few most likely possibilities. The examination also may provide clues as to whether regurgitation is acute or chronic in duration. When transthoracic echocardiographic (TTE) images are not diagnostic for evaluation of mitral valve anatomy and the etiology of regurgitation, transesophageal echocardiographic (TEE) imaging could be helpful [2].

Table 1. Causes of Mitral Regurgitation

Causes of Mitral regurgitation		
Subvalvular apparatus	**Annulus**	**Leaflets**
Ischemic PM dysfunction Calcification Chordal rupture Parachute mitral valve (Shone's complex)	Dilated cardiomyopathy Marfan, Ehlers-Danlos, Pseudoxanthomaelasticum Ischemic Annular dysfunction Mitral annular calcification	Mitral Valve Prolapse Rheumatic valve disease Infective Endocarditis Hypertrophic obstructive cardiomyopathy (HOCM)

TWO DIMENSIONAL ECHOCARDIOGRAM (2D)

Assessment of MR Using 2D echocardiogram

Dysfunction or altered anatomy of any one of the MV components can result in MR (Table 1). Annular dilation may be due to either LA or LV dilation and results in MR because of incomplete leaflet coaptation. The normal mitral apparatus is a saddle-shaped ellipse with its most apical points seen in the apical four-chamber view and its most basal points seen in the long-axis view. Increased rigidity of the annulus, as seen with mitral annular calcification (MAC), impairs systolic contraction of the annulus leading to MR. MAC has a typical appearance on 2D imaging as an area of increased echogenicity on the LA side of the annulus immediately adjacent to the attachment point of the posterior leaflet [4]. Acoustic shadowing, due to the presence of calcium, is seen. In short-axis views the annular calcium may be focal or extensive, involving the entire U-shaped posterior annulus. The region of anterior mitral leaflet–posterior aortic wall continuity is rarely involved. MAC is commonly seen in elderly subjects and in younger patients with renal failure or hypertension (figure 1)

Diseases of the MV leaflets include myxomatous disease, rheumatic disease, endocarditis, Marfan syndrome, and rare disorders such as infiltrative diseases (amyloid, sarcoidosis) and systemic inflammatory disorders (systemic lupus erythematosus, rheumatoid arthritis). Myxomatous MV disease is characterized by thickened, redundant leaflets and chordae with excessive motion and sagging of portions of the leaflets into the LA in systole. The severity of disease is variable, ranging from MV prolapse, in which there is only minimal displacement of the leaflets into the LA in systole, to severe involvement of both leaflets by myxomatous disease with frankly prolapsed or flail leaflet segments (Figure 2). Chordal disruption or elongation leads to MR because of inadequate tensile support of the closed leaflets in systole. With chordal rupture there is a flail segment of the leaflet such that the leaflet is displaced into the LA in systole, with the tip of the leaflet pointing away from the ventricular apex (figure 3).

Endocarditis results in MR by leaflet destruction, perforation, or deformity. Marfan syndrome is associated with a long redundant anterior leaflet that sags into the LA in systole. Infiltrative diseases result in irregular leaflet thickening and inadequate coaptation. Age-related degenerative changes in the mitral leaflets often are seen (with or without associated MAC) and appear as irregular areas of thickening and increased echogenicity of the mitral leaflets

Ischemic MR may be due to regional LV dysfunction with abnormal contraction of the papillary muscle or underlying ventricular wall [5]. Ischemic MR is characterized by restricted leaflet motion, resulting in the appearance of “tenting” or tethering of the mitral valve in systole, which is more pronounced at P3 segment of the MV. In patients with normal resting myocardial function but inducible ischemia with stress, MR may be intermittent.

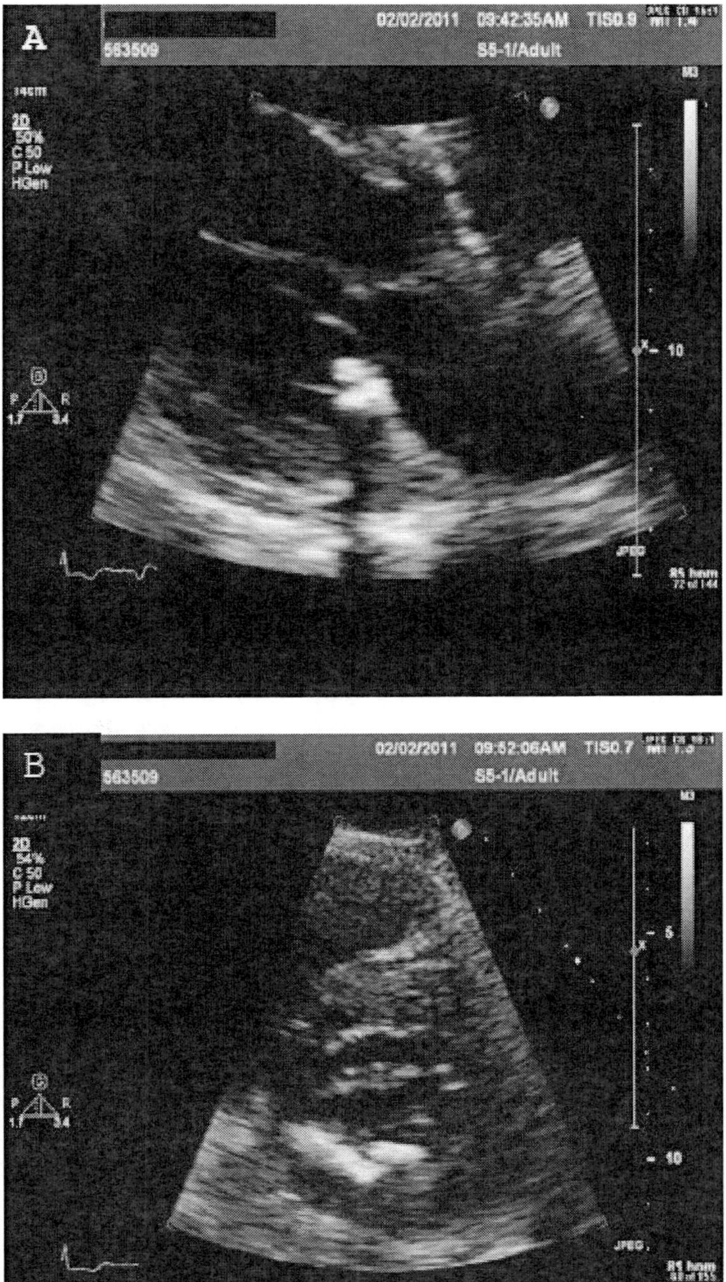

Figure 1. Mitral Annular Calcification (MAC), A) Long access view, B) Short access view.

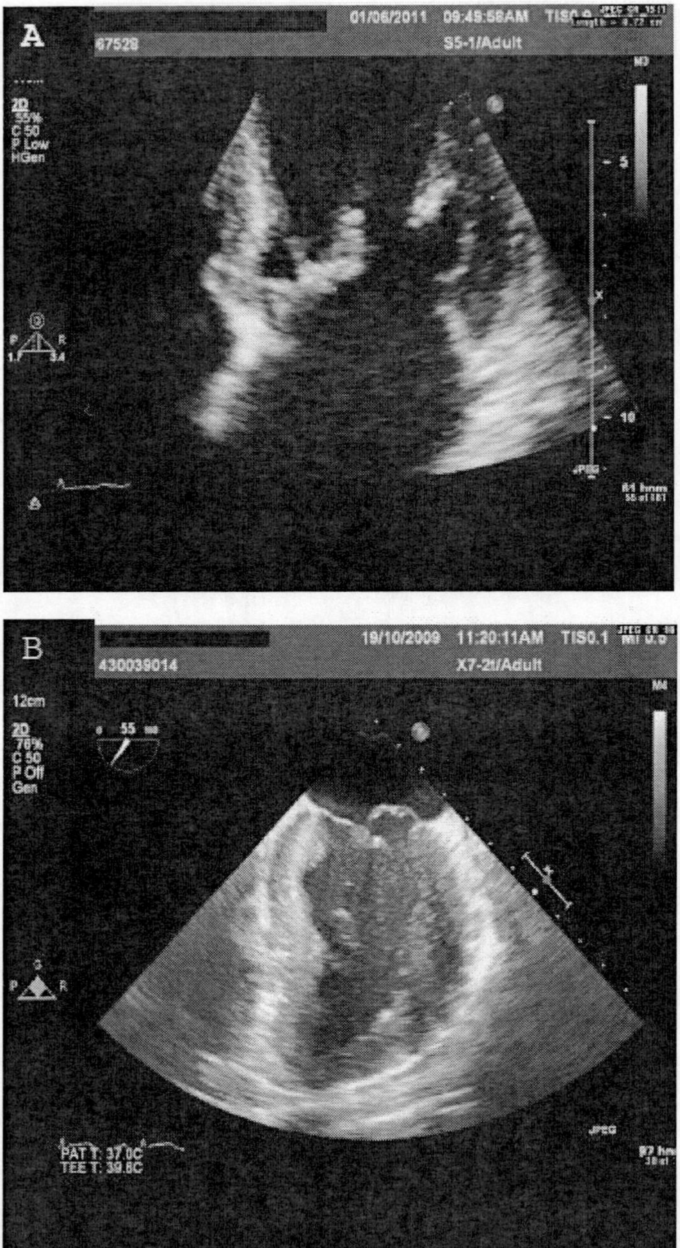

Figure 2. Myxomatous mitral valve disease. A) Showing thickened valve leaflets. B) Excessive tissue with bileaflet prolapse with bowing of the leaflets into LA.

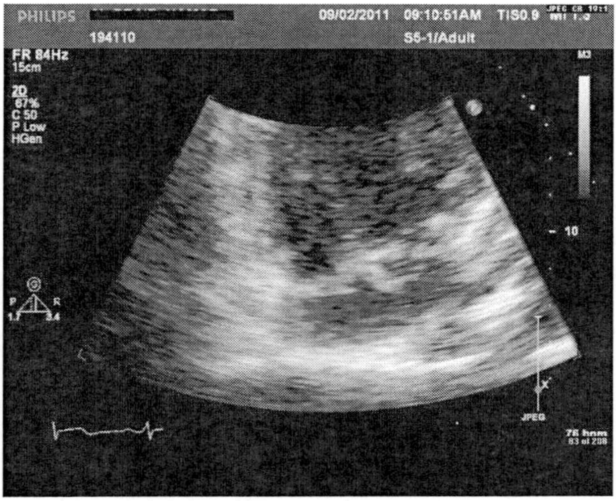

Figure 3. Displacement of mitral leaflet into the LA during systole with a ruptured chordae.

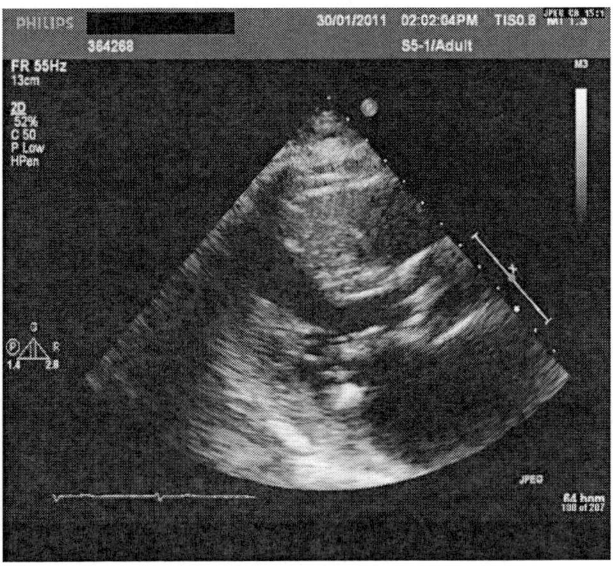

Figure 4. Rheumatic mitral stenosis with thickened leaflets.

Rheumatic MR, like rheumatic mitral stenosis, is characterized by some degree of commissural fusion but chordal fusion and shortening are more prominent (figure 4).

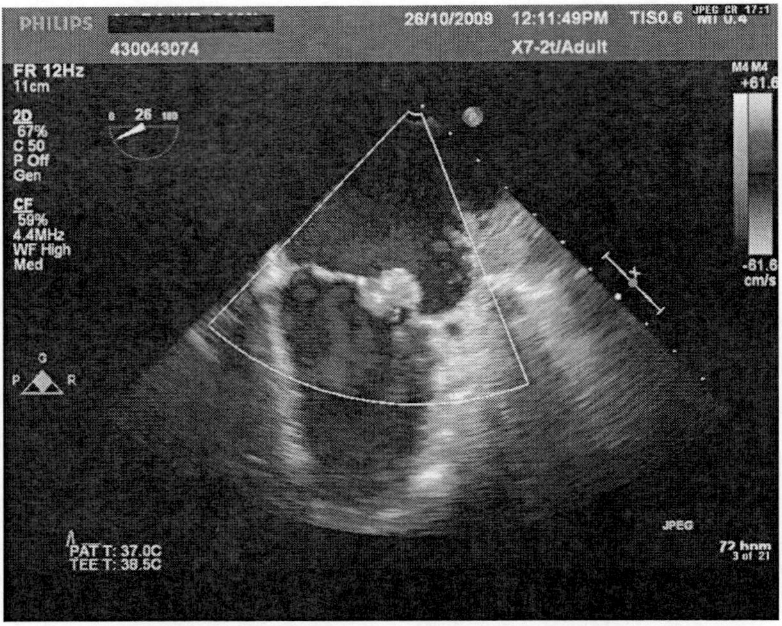

Figure 5. Ruptured head of papillary muscle protruding into the LA during systole.

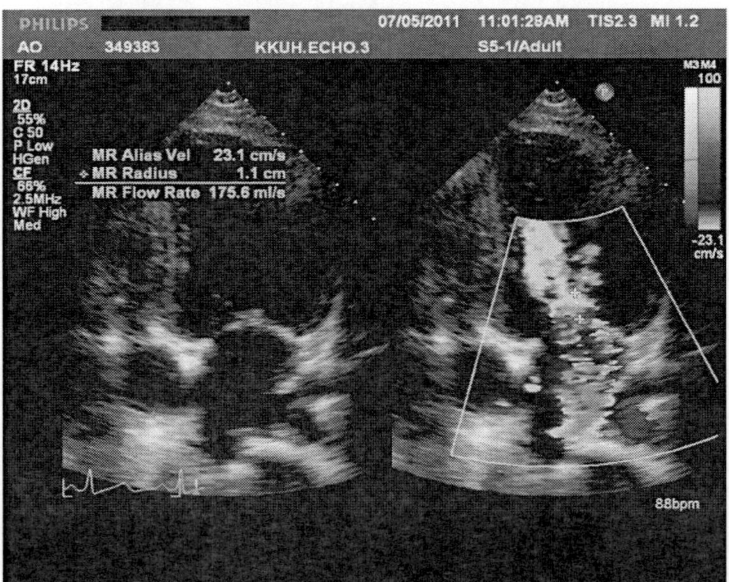

Figure 6. Proximal Isovelocity Surface Area (PISA).

Papillary muscle rupture can occur as a complication of acute myocardial infarction. If the entire papillary muscle is disconnected from the underlying LV wall, few patients survive due to acute severe mitral regurgitation. Echocardiographic evaluation in those who do survive shows a mass (the ruptured papillary muscle) (figure 5) attached to flail segments of anterior and posterior leaflets. The ruptured papillary muscle head is seen in the LA in systole and in the LV in diastole. Severe mitral regurgitation is present on Doppler examination. Partial rupture of a papillary muscle, defined as rupture of one of several "heads" or as partial disconnection of the base of the papillary muscle, is seen more often than complete rupture, as patients are more likely to survive long enough to undergo diagnostic evaluation. In this situation the echocardiogram shows a thin, attenuated, excessively mobile papillary muscle and, if one head has ruptured, a mass attached to the leaflet with prolapse into the LA in systole.

MR due to LV dilation and systolic dysfunction, in patients with normal valve leaflets and chordae, often is called functional MR. The mechanism of functional MR remains unclear. Some studies suggested abnormal orientation of the papillary muscles and/ or annular dilatation [6]. In some cases, it is difficult to determine if MR is the cause or consequence of ventricular dilation and systolic dysfunction. When etiology is unclear, the echocardiographer can describe the valve anatomy and indicate possible reasons for the findings even though the specific tissue diagnosis remains unknown.

Physiologic Consequences of Chronic MR

- Increased LV preload
- Increased stroke volume (SV) secondary to Frank-Starling
- Increased SV force balanced by after-load reduction to LA, normalizing wall stress at cost of elevated LA pressures
- LA pressures reduced chronically by LA dilation
- LV dilation secondary to volume over load
- Eccentric hypertrophy balances LaPlace's law (WT = Pressure x Radius/2T)Systolic function maintained (hyperdynamic) with maintenance of normal forward cardiac output (CO). This mechanism allows chronic MR to be an insidious and well tolerated condition. Decompensation marks the inability of hypertrophy to balance the increase in stroke work, leading to systolic dysfunction.

Evaluation of MR Severity Using 2D Echocardiogram

Initial examination for MR includes color flow imaging and CW Doppler ultrasound. Color Doppler imaging allows detection of the presence of MR and separates mild regurgitation from moderate to severe disease by ultrasound [4, 7, 8] (table 2).

The CW Doppler spectral recording of MR shows a rapid increase in velocity during isovolumic contraction (proportional to the rate of rise in LV pressure or *dP/dt*) from baseline to a maximum velocity of 5 to 6 m/s. The velocity stays high throughout systole with a curve paralleling the rise and fall of LV pressure given a normal LA pressure. During isovolumic relaxation the velocity rapidly returns to baseline. Signal intensity of the MR signal, in comparison with antegrade flow, is related to MR severity. In addition, significant regurgitation is associated with an increase in the antegrade velocity due to increased transmitral volume flow.

With acute MR (table 3), an increase in LA pressure during late systole may be present due to a steep pressure-volume relationship of the nondilated LA. In this situation, the pressure gradient between the LV and the LA is high initially but then begins to equalize in late systole as LA pressure rises. The corresponding Doppler velocity curve shows a high initial velocity with a more rapid fall in velocity in mid- to late systole. This pattern of Doppler velocities also is termed a "v-wave cut off sign"

Table 2. Assessment of severity of mitral valve regurgitation

Severity			Echo parameter
Severe	**Moderate**	**Mild**	
> 10	4-10	< 4	Regurgitant jet area (cm2)
> 40	20-40	< 20	Regurgitant jet fraction (% LA)
> 7	3-7	< 3	Vena Contracta (VC) (mm)
> 0.4	0.2-0.4	< 0.2	Effective regurgitant orifice (ERO) (cm2)
> 60	30-60	< 30	Regurgitant volume (RV) (cc)
> 50	30-50	< 30	Regurgitant fraction (RF) (%)
> 1.2	1-1.2	< 1	Peak E wave velocity (m/sec)
Systolic blunted/ Reversed	Systolic blunted	Normal	Pulmonary venous flow

Table 3. Chronic versus Acute Mitral Regurgitation

Acute	**Chronic**	
Endocarditis Papillary muscle rupture	Myxomatous Ischemic Rheumatic	Etiology
Chordal rupture Papillary muscle rupture Leaflet perforation	Leaflet prolapse Flail leaflet Annular dilation Leaflet restriction	Mechanism
Normal	Normal/ Dilated	LV size
Hyperdynamic	Early: Hyperdynamic Late: Normal/ Depressed	LV systolic function
Normal	Enlarged	LA size
Late-systolic velocity decline ("v-wave cut off sign")	High velocity throughout systole	CW Doppler

A-Vena Contracta (VC)

The vena contracta, the narrowest diameter of the flow stream, reflects the diameter of the regurgitant orifice with the advantages that it is independent of volume flow rate and driving pressure, and it is relatively unaffected by instrument settings. In order to optimize both temporal and spatial resolution [9], the recommended approach to measurement of vena contracta is to use a view that is: 1) perpendicular to jet width, 2) in zoom mode, 3) using narrow sector and 4) have minimal depth. Vena contracta diameter should be measured if color Doppler imaging shows an eccentric or a large jet or if CW Doppler suggests more than mild MR. In patients with MR, vena contracta width is optimally visualized in a parasternal long-axis view, although apical four-chamber and long-axis views may be used if parasternal images are inadequate. The apical two-chamber view is not reliable because the jet width may be broad in this image plane, even though regurgitation is not severe. Vena contracta width also can be measured with TEE imaging. A vena contracta width >0.3 cm indicates that further quantification of regurgitant severity is needed [8, 9].

B-Proximal Isovelocity Surface Area (PISA)

With a central regurgitant jet, regurgitant volume and orifice area can be calculated by the PISA approach. The PISA is optimally imaged in an apical four-chamber view using a narrow sector, minimal depth, and zoom mode.

The PISA also can be imaged from a TEE approach. The aliasing velocity is adjusted to provide a clearly identified hemispherical PISA (figure 6); typically at a velocity limit of 20 to 40 cm/s. Instantaneous regurgitant volume flow rate is calculated. The maximum velocity of the MR-jet on CW Doppler recording is then used to determine regurgitant orifice area (ROA) (figure 7).

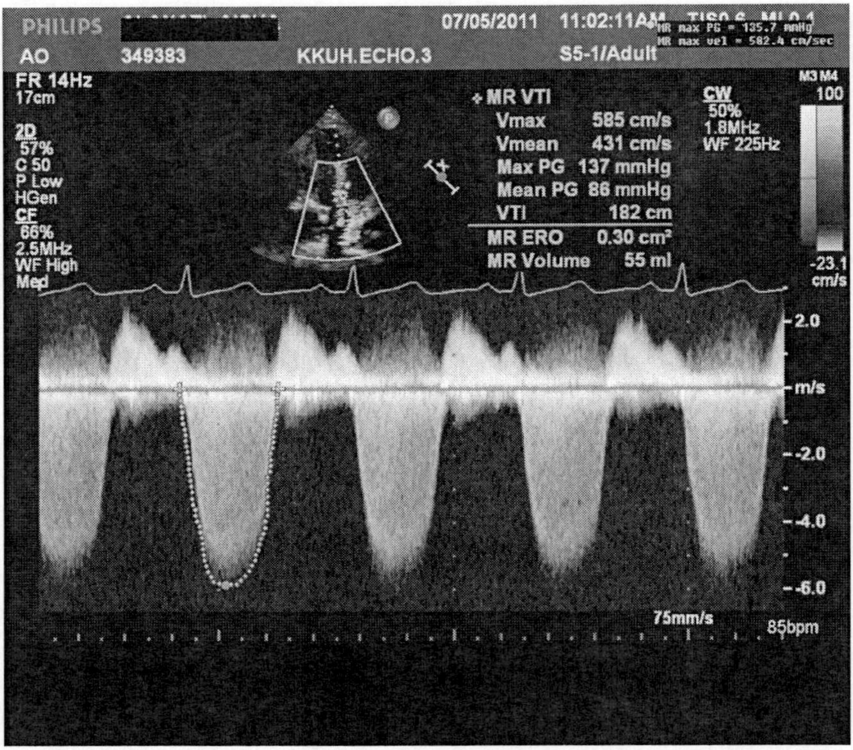

Figure 7. Measuring ROA using the maximum velocity of the MR-jet on CW Doppler recording.

Color flow imaging allows calculation of the retrograde volume flow rate based on measurement of the flow convergence region proximal to the regurgitant orifice. Acceleration of flow occurs proximal to the valve plane with, conceptually, a series of isovelocity "surfaces" leading to the high-velocity jet in the regurgitant orifice. Immediately adjacent to the orifice, these surfaces are small with higher flow velocities; at increasing distances from the orifice, areas are larger, and velocities are lower [10].

The velocity of the PISA can be determined from the color flow image as the aliasing velocity where a distinct red/blue interface is seen. At this interface the velocity is known, being equivalent to the Nyquist limit on the velocity color scale. The size of the PISA can be maximized to allow more accurate regurgitant flow rate calculations by decreasing the velocity range and/or by shifting the velocity baseline. The shape of the isovelocity surface proximal to a regurgitant valve typically is hemispherical with a tendency toward a hemi-elliptical shape closer to the orifice. Assuming a hemispherical shape, the PISA is calculated from measurements of the distance from the aliasing velocity to the regurgitant orifice as the surface area of a hemisphere: Note that the PISA method for calculating regurgitant volume is analogous to calculation of stroke volume proximal to a stenotic valve. The differences between these approaches are (1) the differing shapes of the proximal velocity stream lines; (2) the use of color flow, rather than pulsed Doppler, to measure velocity at a given location; and (3) the need for temporal averaging when color data from single images are used. The PISA method can be combined with the VTI of CW Doppler flow through the regurgitant orifice to calculate ROA. Instead of averaging PISA over the duration of flow, most clinicians calculate the maximum instantaneous regurgitant orifice area (ROA_{max} in cm^2) based on the maximum regurgitant (R_{FR}) flow rate (in mL/s) combined with maximum MR-jet velocity (V_{MR}) in cm/s [2, 7].

C-Regurgitation Volume (RV) and Orifice Area (ROA)

The PISA approach is less accurate with eccentric jets or when the isovelocity surface area is not hemispherical. In these situations quantification of MR by pulsed Doppler volume flow rates is more appropriate. Mitral regurgitant volume (RV_{mitral}) can be calculated from total LV stroke volume measured across the MV (SV_{mitral}) minus forward stroke volume measured in the LV outflow tract (SV_{LVOT}):

D-Pulmonary Vein Flow Reversal

As the MR-jet enters the LA, it displaces blood that was already in the chamber. When severe regurgitation is present, systolic flow reversal in the pulmonary veins is seen. On TTE the flow pattern in the right inferior pulmonary vein can be recorded from the apical four-chamber view in most patients, although the signal-to-noise ratio may be suboptimal at this depth in some adult patients. On TEE the flow pattern in the pulmonary veins can be recorded at high resolution. Examination of all four pulmonary veins is especially helpful with an eccentric regurgitant jet, since the pattern of systolic flow reversal may not be uniform. False-negative results (i.e., a normal pulmonary vein flow pattern despite severe regurgitation) occur when the LA is severely enlarged and compliant so that all the excess volume is contained in the LA without displacement into the pulmonary veins. False-positive results (i.e., blunted or reversed systolic pulmonary vein flow when regurgitation is not severe) occur when an eccentric jet is directed into a pulmonary vein, causing flow reversal in one particular vein. False-positive results also may be seen in patients who are not in sinus rhythm, because the normal pattern of systolic atrial filling partly depends on the preceding emptying of the atrium due to atrial contraction. Other physiologic factors that affect the atrial inflow patterns include respiratory phase, cardiac rhythm, atrial and venous compliance, ventricular diastolic filling, and age. Thus, while the presence and severity of venous systolic flow reversal is a useful adjunct in evaluation of atrioventricular valve regurgitant severity in patients in sinus rhythm, it is not a pathognomonic finding (Figure 8).

Assessment of Mitral Valve Stenosis (MS) Using 2D Echocardiogram

Echocardiographic assessment of patients with MS includes evaluation of:

1) Valve anatomy, mobility, and calcification
2) Transmitral pressure gradient
3) Valve area using 2D echo planimetry, doppler pressure half-time (T½) and/ or continuity equation.
4) Pulmonary artery pressures
5) Coexisting MR

Pressure Gradients

The mean diastolic transmitral pressure gradient can be determined from the transmitral velocity curve (Figure 9) using the simplified Bernoulli equation. Using this velocity curve, pressure gradients can be calculated with the Bernoulli equation and valve area by the T½ method. Note the well-defined maximal velocity and the clearly defined, linear deceleration slope. An A velocity is seen because sinus rhythm is present. With severe stenosis, the mean pressure gradient may be as high as 20 mm Hg but often is only 5 to 15 mm Hg. The variability in pressure gradients in severe mitral stenosis is due to the dependence of pressure gradients on volume flow rate as well as valve area. Severe mitral stenosis may be associated with a low stroke volume (due to the limitation of LV diastolic filling), resulting in a relatively low mean gradient. If volume flow rate increases, for example, with exercise, an increase in transmitral gradient is seen. As for other types of valvular stenosis, calculation of valve area, considering both pressure gradient and volume flow rate, is helpful in quantification of mitral stenosis severity.

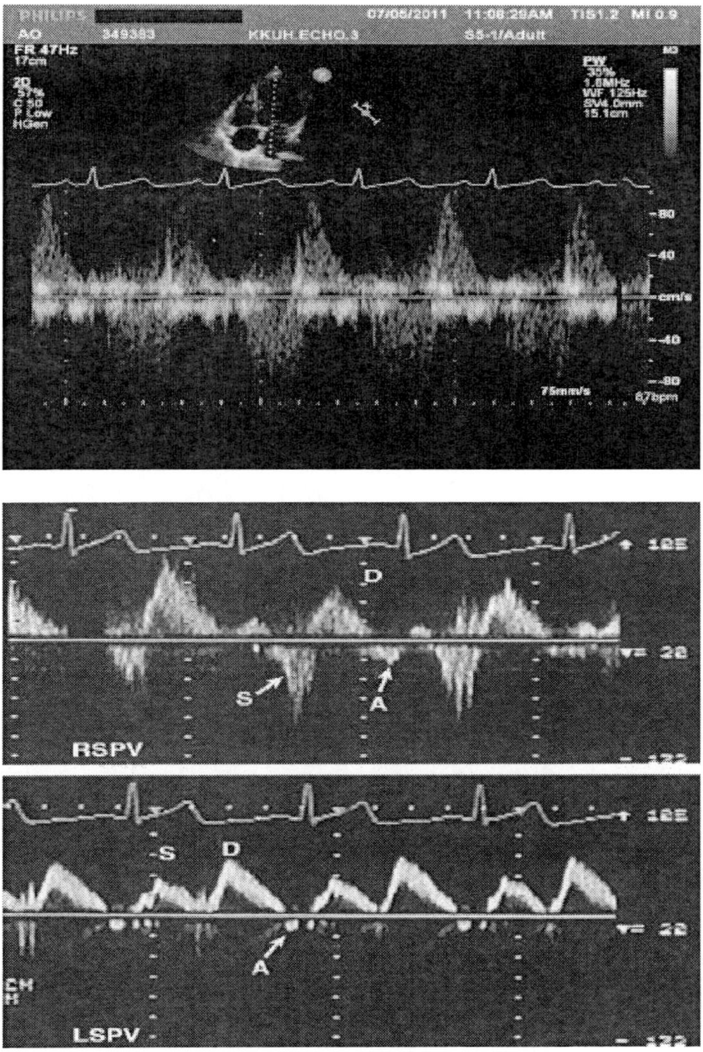

Figure 8. With severe mitral regurgitation, systolic (S) flow reversal in the right superior pulmonary vein (RSPV) Doppler velocity curve (top) and blunting of systolic flow in the left superior pulmonary vein (LSPV) (bottom); A, atrial reversal; D, diastolic flow.

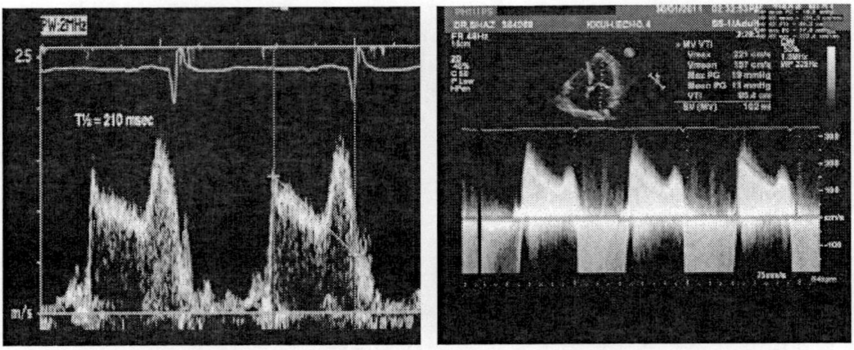

Figure 9. Transmitral flow velocity curve.

Mitral Valve Area

2D Echocardiographic Valve Area by Planimetry

2D short-axis imaging of the diastolic orifice allows direct planimetry of valve area. Because the shape of the MV inflow region is similar to a funnel, with the narrowest opening at the leaflet tips, it is important to begin the 2D scan at the apex, slowly moving the image plane toward the mitral valve to identify the smallest orifice. With a low overall 2D gain setting, the inner edge of the black/white interface is traced. Given the accuracy of this technique, 2D echo mitral valve area (MVA) should be measured in patients with mitral stenosis whenever image quality is adequate [11].

Pressure Half-time (t1/2) Valve Area

Calculation of mitral valve area by the *pressure half-time* (T½) method is based on the concept that the *rate* of pressure decline across the stenotic mitral orifice is determined by the size of the orifice: The smaller the orifice, the slower the rate of pressure decline. The influence of LA and LV compliance on the rate of pressure decline is assumed to be negligible. The pressure half-time is defined as the time interval (in milliseconds) between the maximum early diastolic transmitral pressure gradient and the time point where the pressure gradient is half the maximum value. Initially, this concept was evaluated using invasive measurements of LA and LV pressure, which demonstrated a constant T½ for a given individual, even with exercise-induced changes in volume flow rate, suggesting that this measurement is a constant measure of stenosis severity for a given valve area [12].

This concept then was adapted to transmitral Doppler flow velocity curves. Given the relationship between velocity and pressure gradients, the half-time is determined from a Doppler spectral velocity curve as the time interval from the maximum mitral velocity (V_{max}) to the point where the velocity has fallen by half. Initial studies comparing Doppler half-time data with invasively determined Gorlin valve areas found a linear relationship, with a half-time of approximately 220 ms corresponding to a valve area of 1 cm^2. The empirical formula MVA=220 /T½ was proposed and has been shown to correlate well with invasive valve areas in several clinical studies.

Continuity Equation MV Area

The continuity principle for calculation of valve area also can be applied to the mitral orifice:

MVA=Transmitral SV/VTI MS jet

Table 4. Pitfalls of different methods of measuring MVA

Method of Assessment	Disadvantages
Pressure Gradient	1) Intercept angle between mitral stenosis jet and ultrasound beam 2) Beat-to-beat variability in atrial fibrillation 3) Dependence on transvalvular volume flow rate (e.g., exercise, coexisting mitral regurgitation)
2D Valve Area	1) Image orientation 2) Tomographic plane 3) 2D gain settings 4) Intraobserver and interobserver variability in planimetry of orifice 5) Poor acoustic access 6) Deformed valve anatomy post-valvuloplasty
T½ Valve Area	1) Definition of V_{max} and early-diastolic slope 2) Nonlinear early-diastolic velocity slope 3) Sinus rhythm with *a* wave superimposed on early-diastolic slope 4) Influence of coexisting aortic regurgitation 5) Changing LV and LA compliances immediately after commissurotomy
Continuity Equation	1) Accurate measurement of transmitral stroke volume

Table 5. 3D Echocardiography Protocol

View	Imaging
Parasternal	• Full volume imaging • 3D color doppler of the mitral and aortic valves • 3D color doppler of the tricuspid and pulmonary valves
Apical	• Full volume imaging • Includes both atria and ventricles • 3D color doppler of the mitral, aortic, tricuspid and pulmonary valves
Subcostal	• Full volume imaging • 3D color doppler of the interatroal and interventricular septa
Suprasternal	• Full volume imaging • 3D color doppler at the level of the descending aorta

where SV is stroke volume (cm^3), VTI is the velocity-time integral (cm) in the mitral stenosis jet, and MVA (cm^2) is the mitral valve area. Stroke volume can be determined from the LVOT CSA and VTI (in the absence of aortic or mitral regurgitation). Note that stroke volume measured at either of these sites will represent transmitral volume flow accurately only if there is no significant mitral regurgitation. There are several disadvantages for each of these methods used to assess the severity of mitral valve stenosis (table 4) and its use should be complementary [8, 13].

Common Etiologies of Mitral Valve Stenosis

Rheumatic Disease

Rheumatic disease predominantly affects the mitral valve and is almost always the cause of mitral stenosis. Rheumatic valvular disease is characterized by commissural fusion, which results in bowing or doming of the valve leaflets in diastole (Figure 10). Thickening at the leaflet tips occurs frequently, but the remainder of the leaflets can show variable degrees of thickening and/or calcification [14]. If the base and mid-portions of the leaflets are relatively thin, leaflet mobility is normal other than the fused commissures. The rheumatic process also typically affects the subvalvular region with fusion, shortening, fibrosis, and calcification of the mitral chordae.

MAC is a common finding on echocardiography in elderly subjects. Mild annular calcification appears as an isolated area of calcification on the LA side of the posterior annulus, near the base of the posterior mitral leaflet. In more severe mitral annular calcification, increased echogenicity is seen in a hemi-elliptical pattern involving the entire posterior annulus. Mitral annular calcification may result in mild-to-moderate mitral regurgitation due to increased rigidity of the mitral annulus. Occasionally the calcification extends into the base of the mitral leaflets themselves, rarely resulting in functional mitral stenosis due to narrowing of the diastolic flow area. Calcific mitral stenosis can be distinguished from rheumatic disease by careful imaging techniques to demonstrate thick and mobile mitral leaflet tips without commissural fusion.

THREE-DIMENSIONAL ECHOCARDIOGRAM (3D)

History and Development of 3D Echocardiogram

The term *3D echocardiography* refers broadly to several approaches for acquisition and display of cardiac ultrasound images. Different 3D approaches are similar in that cardiac structures are shown in relationship to each other in all three spatial dimensions and in that structures can be rotated or viewed from different orientations, even after image acquisition. One of the challenges of 3D echocardiography is ensuring adequate image resolution in all three dimensions, given the constraints of ultrasound physics and transducer design. Another challenge is ensuring temporal, as well as spatial resolution [15].

Attempts to record and display ultrasound images in 3D format were first reported in the 1960s. One of the earliest studies described the acquisition of a series of parallel scans of a human orbit to reconstruct 3D anatomy. Despite the limited technology at that time, these initial studies demonstrated that complex anatomic structures were ideally displayed using 3D techniques. Concerns about image quality and the computational power needed for storage and reconstruction greatly limited the early application of this methodology. More than a decade later, investigators began to obtain 3D ultrasound images of the heart. Through the careful tracking of a transducer, a sequence of 2D echocardiograms could be recorded, aligned, and reconstructed into a 3D data set. This methodology was limited by the need for offline data processing to create and display the 3D images. In the early 1990s, von Ramm and colleagues developed the first real-time 3D (RT-3D) echocardiographic scanner, capable of acquiring volumetric data at frame rates sufficient to depict cardiac motion. More recently, further improvements in design and engineeering have led to the commercialization of RT-3D echocardiography. This methodology has evolved quickly, and different versions of RT-3D imaging are currently available on several platforms. The advantages of RT-3D TTE have been clearly demonstrated [16], in an effort to advance this technology from the research arena to general clinical practice.

Reconstruction Techniques

Early approaches to 3D echocardiography were based on the principle that a 3D data set could be reconstructed from a series of 2D images. In this method, serial 2D images are obtained using either freehand scanning or a mechanically driven transducer that sequentially recorded images at predefined intervals [17]. With freehand scanning, a series of images are obtained by manually tilting the transduceralong a fixed plane, and a spatial locator attached to the transducer translates the 3D spatial location onto a Cartesian coordinate system. This approach has several practical limitations, including the relative bulk of the acoustic spatial locators, which makes transducer manipulation difficult, and the need for a clear and direct path between the acoustic locators and the transmitter. For electromagnetic spatial locator systems, an additional problem is the potential for interference of the electromagnetic field by ferromagnetic material in close proximity to the transducer (e.g. material in hospital beds and medical equipment). An alternative to freehand scanning is the use of a mechanized transducer to obtain serial images at set intervals in a parallel fashion or by pivoting around a fixed axis in a rotational, fanlike manner. Because the intervals and angles between the 2D images are defined, a 3D coordinate system can be derived from the 2D images in which the volume is more uniformly sampled than with the freehand scanning approach.

More recently, the use of a transesophageal or transthoracic multiplane probe has emerged as areadily available method to obtain rotational images at defined interval angles around a fixed axis. Typically, 10-15 images are collected over a 180-degree rotation at set intervals. To minimize reconstruction artifacts, sequential images are gated to both electrocardiography (ECG) and respiration. The acquisition of a complete data set typically takes 1 to 5 minutes, depending on respiratory and heart rates and thepredefined spatial intervals. During cardiac surgery, respiration can be suspended during acquisition to minimize the effects of respiratory motion. The quality of 3D reconstructions from 2D images depends on a number of factors, including the intrinsic quality of the ultrasound images, the number (or density) of the 2D images used to reconstruct the 3D image, the ability to limit motion artifact, and adequate ECG and respiratory gating. In general, the greater the number of images obtained (ie, the smaller the space intervals between images), the better the 3D reconstruction. However, increasing the number of images also lengthens the acquisition time, which can potentially introduce motion artifact. Consequently, the optimal number of images necessary for 3D reconstruction depends on the cardiac structure being examined and the resolution required. For example, 4 to 6 serial images are usually adequate for volume reconstructions ofthe LV, whereas more images are often needed to visualize more complex, rapidlymoving structures, such as mitral and aortic valves [18]. Once the 2D images have been obtained, they are processed offline with customized or commercially available software. The cardiac structures are manually or semi-automatically traced to the 3D spatial coordinates to reconstruct a 3D image

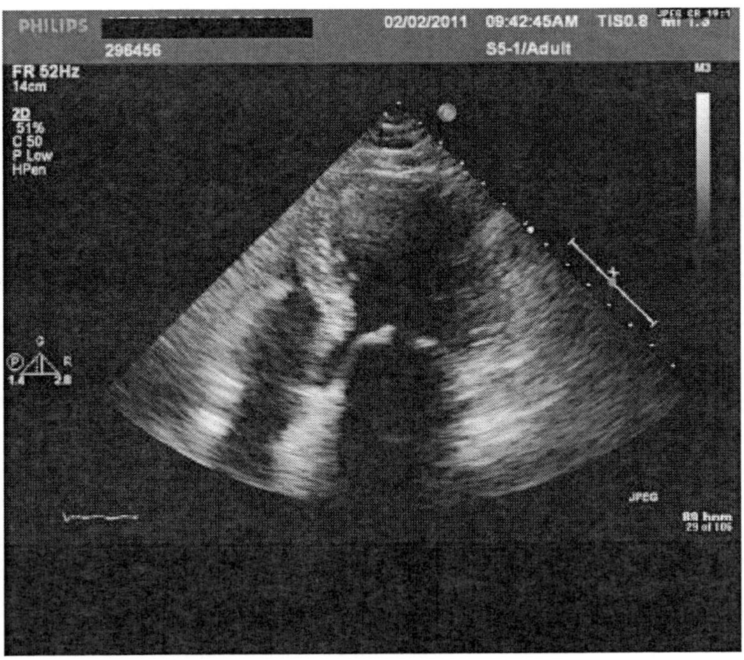

Figure 10. Bowing of the valve leaflets in diastole in rheumatic valve.

Real-Time 3D Acquisition Methods

Several studies [17-22] have demonstrated that 3D reconstruction from serial 2D images provides accurate anatomic information suitable for quantitative analysis. However, this methodology is subject to technical limitations during image acquisition and requires significant offline data processing. The development of RT3D echocardiographic systems circumvents many of the disadvantages of reconstructive methods. RT3D echocardiography uses a transducer with ultrasound elements arranged in a grid fashion. The earliest devices, developed by von Ramm and colleagues, used a sparse-array matrix transducer transmitting at a frequency of 2.5 or 3.5 MHz. These transducers consisted of 256 non simultaneous firing elements and acquired a pyramidal volume data set measuring 60° X 60° within a single heartbeat. However, the resolution and image quality of this first-generation sparse-array transducer were relatively poor and often inferior to standard 2D images; frame rates were low; and the pyramidal volume had a narrow sector angle of 60°, resulting in an inability to accommodate larger ventricles. Moreover, the images obtained with this system were not volume-rendered online; instead, they consisted of computer-generated 2D cut planes derived from the 3D volume data set. These features limited clinical application of this pioneering technology. Current RT3D systems use matrix-array transducer technology with a greater number of imaging elements, typically containing more than 3000 imaging elements, compared with the 256 in the sparse-array transducer. These current matrix-array transducers offer improved resolution and are rapidly becoming the primary technique for 3D data acquisition in clinical and research practice. However, recent improvements in transducer technology have resulted in [1] a smaller transducer footprint, improved side-lobe suppression, greater sensitivity and penetration, and harmonic capabilities that may be used for both gray-scale and contrast imaging. In addition, these matrix-array transducers display either online 3D volume-rendered images or 2 to 3 simultaneous orthogonal 2D imaging planes (i.e. biplane or triplane imaging). RT3D systems generally have 3 acquisition modes: real time (narrow), zoom (magnified), and wide angle. The real-time mode displays a pyramidal data set of approximately 50° X 30°. The zoom mode displays a smaller, magnified pyramidal data set of 30° X 30° at a higher resolution. The wide-angle mode provides a pyramidal data set of approximately 90° X 90°, which allows inclusion of a larger cardiac volume. This wide-angle mode requires ECG gating, because the wide-angle data set is compiled by merging 4 narrower pyramidal scans obtained over 4 consecutive heartbeats. To minimize reconstruction artifacts, data should be acquired during suspended respiration if possible. Although wideangle data sets provide a larger pyramidal scan, this is at the cost of lower resolution, which is decreased compared with the narrow-angle 3D mode. Once a 3D data set is acquired, it must be sliced or "cropped" to visualize the cardiac structures within the pyramid. Multiple cropping methods are available, but a common method displays 2 or 3 imaging planes simultaneously. Each of these imaging planes can be manipulated separately to appropriately align the cardiac structures. Another cropping method involves a single-slice plane that can be manually adjusted to expose and display the cardiac structures of interest

3D TEE Protocol to Evaluate the Mitral Valve

A complete 3D echocardiographic study includes an assessment of ventricular function, valvular morphology, and hemodynamic status. Unlike 2D echocardiography, in which standard views are described based on the plane through which they pass, 3D echocardiography is inherently volumetric. As such, it permits both an external view of the heart and multiple internal perspectives (through cropping). A general approach is to describe cardiac structures using both the ultrasoundplane and the viewing perspective. Three orthogonal planes are recommended [21, 23]: (1) the sagittalplane, which corresponds to a vertical, long axis view of the heart; (2) the coronal plane, which corresponds to a 4-chamber view; and (3) the transverse plane, which corresponds to a short-axis view. Each plane can be viewed from 2 sides, which represent opposite perspectives; for example, the transverse plane, which represents the short-axis view, can be visualized from the perspective of the apex or base; the coronal plane can be viewed from above or below; and the sagittal plane can be viewed from the left or right. The choice of narrow-angle or wide-angle imaging acquisition modes depends on the cardiac structure to be examined. For imaging of the ventricles, it is best to use a wide-angle acquisition in the apical window (4-chamber) so as to include the entire ventricle. For smaller structures, such as the aortic valve, anarrow-angle acquisition may be adequate for the cardiac structure to be examined.

As an alternative to a complete 3D study, 3D echocardiography can be performed selectively as a complement to a 2D study. For example, in apatient with mitral stenosis, the 3D portion of the study may be limited to visualization and quantificationof the mitral orifice. Focused 3D imaging for LV volume calculation, typically performed with an apical 4-chamber wide-angle acquisition, also can be used to complement standard 2D imaging. The ability to extract hemodynamic information derived from 3D color Doppler ultrasonography is currently being investigated. To capture and analyze color flow imaging in 3 dimensions, the area of interest should be obtained within the 3D data set, with the angle of the ultrasound beam aligned as parallel as possible to the direction of blood flow. Depth and sector settings should be optimized for color Doppler resolution. Extraneous flows can be cropped so that only the area of interest is displayed. The color Doppler flow patterns can be analyzed in multiple views to provide a complete assessment of the color Doppler data (Figure 11) (table 5).

Table 6. Three-dimensional transesophageal echocardiographic protocol to evaluate the mitral valve

Protocol	Primary Objectives	Secondary Objectives	Special Applications
Simultaneous Biplane	Image and plane optimization, LV size & function, LA size, presence and severity of MR	Spectral Doppler readings, peak & mean MV gradients, MV area by pressure t1/2, pulmonary veins flow reversal	Structural heart disease interventions, inter-atrial septal puncture, guidance for position & delivery of devices
Large Sector	Registration of LV, LA and MV for post-processing analysis	Comprehensive cardiac morphology assessment, 3D MR volumes	Dyssynchrony evaluation, segmental LV wall motion analysis
Narrow Sector	Characterization of leaflets, commissures, MV orifice and Chordae	Characterization of LAA	Guidance of catheters & devices during Structural heart disease interventions
Wide Sector Focused	Characterization of MV apparatus	Characterization of LAA and pulmonary veins	Guidance of catheters & devices during Structural heart disease interventions

Table 7. Strengths & Weaknesses of 3D Echocarduiography

Strengths	Weaknesses
1) Inclusion of the whole heart within a data set allows for correction of foreshortening 2) Rapid on-line direct volumetric analysis with no need for geometric assumptions 3) Great accuracy for LV mass, volumes and EF when compared to MRI. 4) Improved iter-, intra- and test-retest variability 5) Regional volumetric analysis capabilities. 6) Improved anatomical assessment of valves 7) Similar excellent safety profile 8) Ability to obtain global and regional data from one analysis (volumes, EF and dyssynchrony)	1) Additional training and software required 2) 2D imaging from 3D transducers is currently not as good as for dedicated 2D probes 3) Reduced temporal and spatial resolution 4) Not currently as widely available as 2D imaging 5) Not yet fully integrated with data storage systems used for 2D echo 6) " Stitching" artefacts, particularly in those with significant arrhythmias 7) Not fully incorporated into major society guidelines 8) Differences in data derived from different software packages need to be further delineated

There is already a substantial body of literature demonstrating the added value of 3D over 2D echocardiography in the evaluation of patients with mitral valve disease.9,15-25 Real-time 3D TEE provides a more authentic representation of the mitral valve structure, function, and pathology compared with traditional 2D and 3D TTE. The spatial relationships of the components of the mitral valve complex are facilitated by the use of 3DTEE. The following protocol for 3D TEE provides a comprehensive evaluation of the mitral valve apparatus (figure 12) (table 6).

Simultaneous Biplane Format

Simultaneous longitudinal biplane images of the mitral valve are obtained in multiple angles. With a reference 4-chamber plane set at 0 to 20 degrees, multiple recordings for the second plane are registered in30 degrees intervals from 30 to 150 degrees. This is done with and without color Doppler.

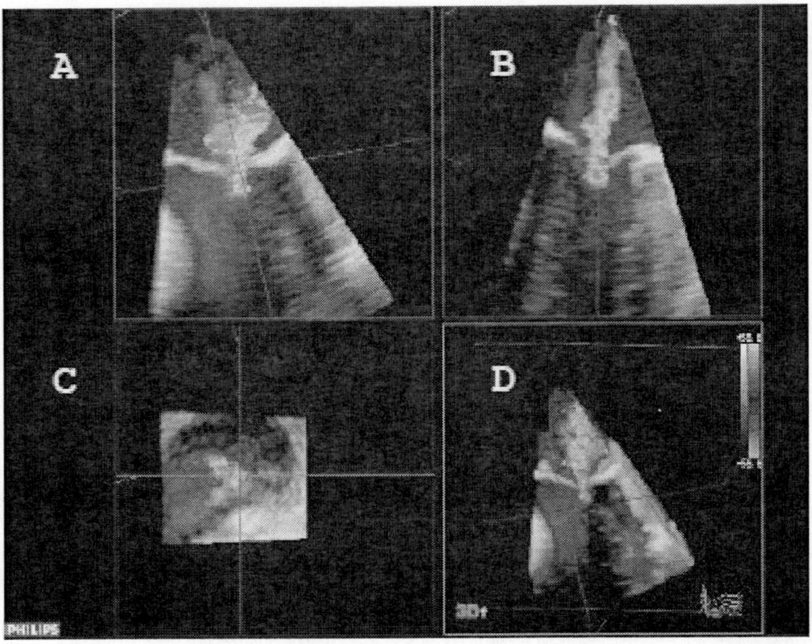

Figure 11. 3D color Doppler display of mitral regurgitation. A) Coronal, B) Sagittal, C) Transverse, D) Full Volume.

Large-Sector Format

After optimizing the position of the mitral valve using the biplane format, large-sector data sets with and without color Doppler are obtained. After confirming that the mitral apparatus, the left ventricle, and the floor of the left atrium are included, the images are stored for review. Care is taken to minimize ''stitching'' artifacts by avoidingprobe motion, premature contractions, and marked respiratory changes during image acquisition.

Narrow-Sector Format

Keeping the transesophageal echocardiographic probe in the mid-esophagus, 3D narrow-sector images equivalent to the 4-chamber 2-chamber, and 3-chamber views on 2D TEE are displayed and recorded. The narrow sector usually does not permit full visualization of the mitral valve, so it is necessary to rotate the image to see the valve from all perspectives. We have found that a bicommissural view registered at 60 degrees includes most of the mitral valve leaflets. Different levels of anterior and posterior tilt and elevation are applied to optimize the visual plane.

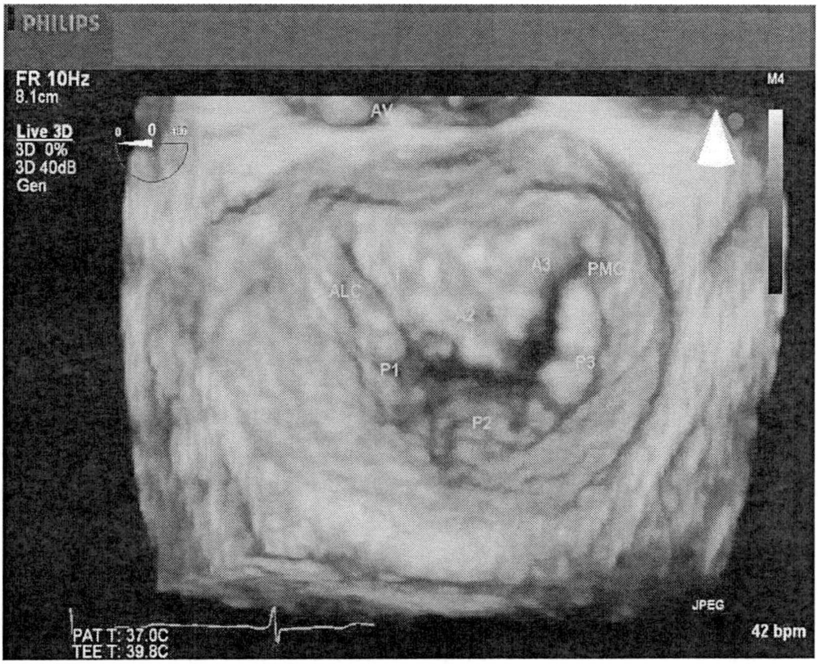

Figure 12. Wide-sector focused 3D TEE of a normal mitral valve. Mitral valve as seen from the left atrium. The ''surgeon's view'' with the aortic valve (AV) at the 12 o'clock position is presented. The segments of the anterior (A1, A2, and A3) and posterior (P1, P2, and P3) leaflet are clearly identified. The anterolateralcommissure (ALC) is clearly seen between the A1 and P1 segments. The posteromedialcommissure (PMC) is clearly seen between the A3 and P3 segments.

Wide-Sector Focused Format

A truncated pyramidal data set is obtained by selecting a region of interest that includes the mitral valve, the aortic valve, and the left atrial appendage. The initial presentation of this tomographic slice is seen from its side and provides no morphologic information. This crosssectional ultrasound data set needs to be tilted downwards to visualize the mitralvalve. The aortic valve is used as reference, and when rotated to about 12 o'clock on an imaginary clock face, one obtains an anatomic view of the mitral valve with a perspective similar to that observed by a cardiac surgeon inspecting the mitral valve from the left atrium. The lateral aspect of the MV represented by left atrial appendage, is visualized on the left side of the screen. By tilting the image 180, the mitral valve is inspected from its ventricular surface.

Morphologic Assessment of the MV by 3D TEE

Three-dimensional echocardiography is the diagnostic technique that has contributed most toour knowledge of MV anatomy and function [23-25]. Through in vitro studies and 3D studies conducted in animal models, changes that occur in mitral and ventricular geometry following myocardialinfarction, thereby giving rise to MR, have been demonstrated.8 Later studies in patients confirmed these results and most have focused on functional MR (FMR) due to its complex underlying mechanism. In FMR, the MV is apparently structurally normal. There is an imbalance between the closing forces on the MV during systole. On one hand, due to ventricular dysfunction and diminished contractility, there is a consequent reduction in closing force on the MV. On the other hand, apical and lateral papillary muscle (PM) displacement, secondary to adverse LV remodeling, causes apically- directed traction of the mitral leaflets, reduces the degree of MV coaptation, and results in MR. Moreover, the mitral annulus usually dilates to a greater degree. Using 3D TEE, we can analyze the components of the mitral apparatus in detail, thereby understanding normal functional anatomy and the changes that occur in FMR. A systematic evaluation of the MV complex includes a detailed analysis of all of its components. In the following, we summarize the use of 3DTEE for the detailed analysis of the MV apparatus

Mitral Annulus

Mitral annular non-planarity during systole has been documented on 3D TTE by Levine et al. It has been demonstrated by 3D TTE that the mitral annulus and leaflets have a saddle-shaped contour (a hyperbolic-paraboloid); this explains the apparent prolapse of the mitral valve in the apical 4-chamber view in some normal individuals. It has also been demonstrated that there is flattening of the mitral annulus during dilatation of the LV, with resultant FMR. The increased analytic detail possible with 3DTEE is likely to further clarify mitral annular geometry and the changes in size and shape that occur during the cardiac cycle. In addition, the characteristics of the mitral annulus in patients fitted with annuloplastyrings have been characterized by 3D TTE; the improved spatial resolution of 3D TEE will only enhance our capacity to evaluate the mitral annulus in patients being considered for mitral repair with annuloplasty surgery. MV annular geometry and function can be evaluated using 3DTEE by the use of serial cropping of the large-sector data set until the circumference of the annulus is found. For a true 3D rendition of the MV annulus, offline 3D processing is required. 3D modeling software is used to trace the contour of the MV leaflets and annulus, with resulting representative images of the 3D morphology of the mitral annulus. Through these reconstructions, it is now possible to measure the annular circumference, annular major and minor diameters, and annular height.

MV Leaflets

The anterior and posterior MV leaflets can be visualized with great detail with the 3D TEE formats. The wide-angle format is preferred for a global visualization of the mitralleaflets and adjacent structures. The large-sector focused format provides the best anatomic characterization of the mitral leaflets. The MV can be seen from the LA and LV perspective. When using the LA perspective, the anterior mitral leaflet obliterates approximately two thirds ofthe anterior aspect of the mitral orifice during systole extending from the aorto-mitral fibrosa and left and right fibrous trigones to the line of coaptation. Systolic bulging of the central aspect of the anterior leaflet toward the LA can frequently be appreciated. The posterior mitral leaflet is seen extending from the anterolateral to the posteromedialcommissures, semi-encircling the anterior leaflet and obliterating the posterior third of the mitral orifice. The anterolateral (P1), middle (P2), and posteromedial (P3) scallops can beeasily discerned. These en face views of the MV permit clear characterization of MV prolapse and flail MV segments (Figure 13).

A detailed analysis of the MV commissures is of particular interest in patients being considered for MV balloon valvuloplasty. The anterolateral commisure is next to the left fibrous trigoneand the left atrial appendage; the posteromedial commisure is next to the right fibrous trigone and the interatrial septum. The commissures can be best explored from the mid-esophageal position by 3D TEE with the real-time narrow format, which has the best temporal and spatial resolution. Each commisure is inspected from the left atrium and left ventricle. The presence and degree of commissural fusion and the severity of calcification are noted. The high-resolution images of the mitral leaflets obtained with the3D TEE probe allow for detailed characterization of vegetations, flecks of calcium, or thrombotic material on the surface of theMV. In addition, abnormalities of leaflet motion and function such as seen in hypertrophic obstructive cardiomyopathy can be clearly discerned on 3D TEE. During diastole, the leaflets move in the opposite direction, exposing the inflow of the LV. In patients with MS, the funnel-shaped narrowing of the MV can be appreciated from this perspective. From the ventricular perspective, the free borders of the mitral leaflets are seen to coapt during systole and to open during diastole. In patients with MS, commissural fusion can bebest appreciated from this ventricular perspective. In our initial experience, this view has proved most useful in evaluating the immediate results of mitral valve balloon valvuloplasty

Chordae Tendineae

The chordae tendineae play a central role in the normal function of the mitral complex. There are about 120 individual chordae that originate from the tips of the papillary muscles and end in both of the mitral leaflets. The ''primary'' chordae are attached to the free margin or edge of both leaflets; the secondary chordae are attached a few millimeters into the ventricular surface of the leaflets, and the commissural chordae are attached into each commisure. The chordal attachments and the tips of the papillary muscles can be best evaluated with the wide-angle focused format from the LV perspective. However, the best visualization of the mitral subvalvular apparatus is gained from the trans-gastric long-axis viewof the MV and LV; our current practice for evaluating patients with MS is to obtain a narrow-sector image of the subvalvular apparatus, on the long-axis view, in search for chordal shortening and fusion and to evaluate the distance between the papillary muscles and the tip of the mitral leaflets as markers of the degree of subvalvular stenosis.

LV Wall and Papillary Muscles

The role of the papillary muscles and adjacent LV walls as important components of the mitral valve complex is well established. There are usually two papillary muscles that originate as muscular projections between the apex and middle portion of the LV cavity.31 The anterolateral papillary muscle is usually single and originates from the anterolateral LV wall. The posteromedial papillary muscle is usually composed of 2 or 3 muscular groups. The heads of the papillary muscles taper into fibrous projections, giving origin to the chordae tendineae. The papillary muscles can be best visualized and characterized with 3D TEE from the trans-gastric views with the narrow-angle format. 3D TEE would appear ideally suited to characterize abnormalities of the papillary muscles, including fibrosis, necrosis, and rupture. This in our view represents an important area for further studies and investigation. Real-time 3D TEE provides excellent images from which it is possible to assess global as well as segmental LV function in real time.

Through these methods, the potential role of LV wall motion abnormalities or papillary muscle dysfunction on the development and severity of mitral regurgitation can be elucidated. It is also wellestablished that LV mechanical dyssynchrony is a compounding factor in the development and progression of functional mitral regurgitation. 3D TEE permits detailed evaluation of mechanical dyssynchrony, and it is likely to become powerful tool in the evaluation of mitral insufficiency secondary to or aggravated by LV dyssynchrony.

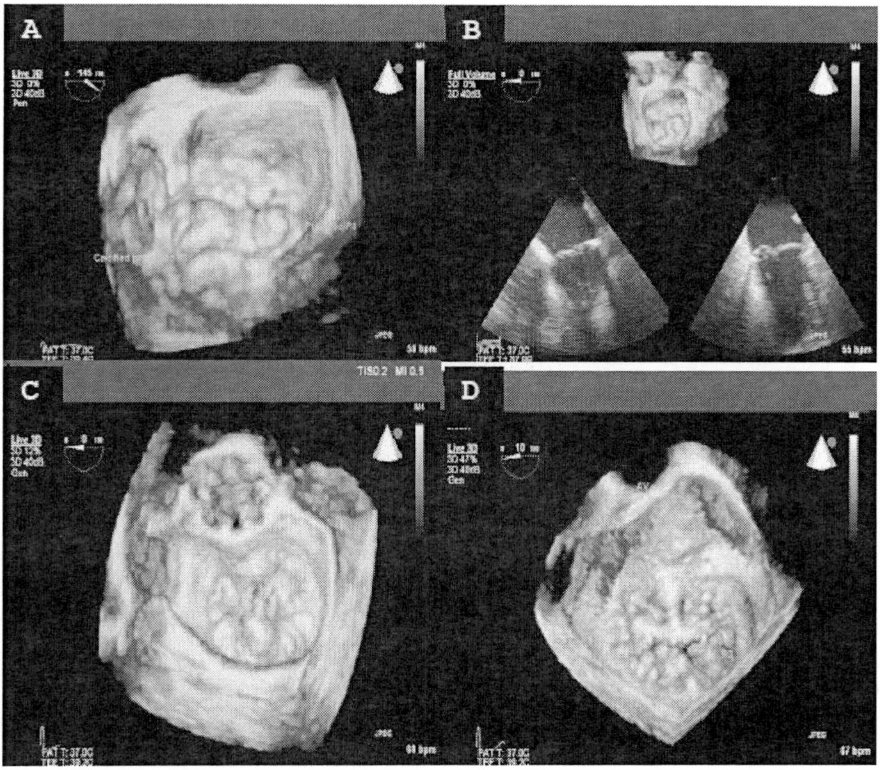

Figure 13. Mitral valve prolapse. A) flail P1, B) prolapsed P1 & P3, C) flail P2, D) prolapsed P3.

LA, Left Atrial Appendage, and Pulmonary Veins

A comprehensive evaluation of the mitral complex includes the assessment of LA size and volume as well as interrogation of adjacent structures, particularly the interatrial septum, left atrial appendage, and pulmonary veins. RT-3D TEE is uniquely suited for this purpose. The mid-esophageal view provides a unique perspective from which the floor and lateral walls of the LA, the LA appendage, and the pulmonary veins can be imaged in great detail. However, the deep trans-gastric 5-chamber view is bettersuited to visualize the entire LA. Therefore, to visualize the lower half of the left atrium, the LA appendage, and the pulmonary veins, we use full-volume or real-time zoom images obtainedfrom the mid-esophagus, whereas to better asses left atrial volume, weuse a deep trans-gastric approach with full-volume 3D format.

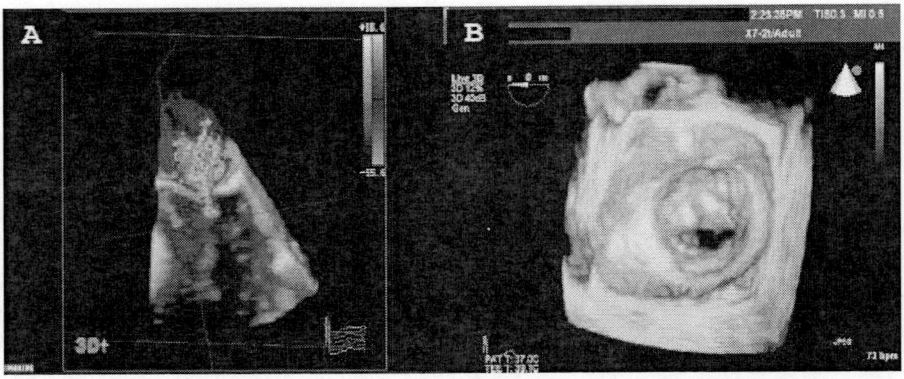

Figure 14. Posterior leaflet restriction. A) full volume color Doppler. B) Wide sector focused 3D image.

Color Doppler 3D TEE

In addition to clearly defining mitral morphology and pathology, 3D TEE, through the use of color Doppler, has the potential to improve the characterization of mitral regurgitant jets and the estimation of mitral regurgitation severity. All the 2D color Doppler quantitative and semi quantitative methods have the potential to be refined with 3D techniques. Sugeng et al reported that 3D TEE of regurgitant jets is feasible in the majority of patients and that it provides additional information to that obtained from2D examinations. In vitro and clinical validation studies with 3D TTE have demonstrated improved accuracy in the estimation of mitral regurgitation severity by directly measuring the proximal isovelocity surface area and vena contracta without geometric assumptions [25, 26]. Color 3DTEE particularly helpful in the analysis of eccentric jets, as more realistic estimates of color jet volumes can be ascertained using the 3D method.

Clinical Applications of 3D Echocardiography of the MV

Assessment of MR

MR is the second most common valvular lesion that ultimately progresses to irreversible left and right-sided heart failure with excess morbidity and mortality. In view of recent advances in MV repair techniques and their early use to preserve ventricular function, timely diagnosis and accurate assessment of severity of MR are of significant importance for appropriate decision making and patient outcome. 2Dechocardiography with color-flow Doppler is currently the standard method for noninvasive assessment of severity and etiology of MR. However, accurate quantitative evaluation of MR severity remains challenging because limited scan plane orientation of 2D echo cardiography does not provide direct measurement of the regurgitant lesion. Although effective regurgitant orifice area (EROA) has been demonstrated to be an important parameter of MR severity and prognosis, determination of EROA by the use of quantitativeDoppler or PISA method is limited because of indirect measurements apart from the lesion itself and multiple computational steps based on inaccurate hemodynamic assumptions [27]. As a practical approach to EROA, the VC width of a color-flow Doppler jet has recently evolved to an accepted semiquantitative parameter for MR severity. This measure corresponds hemodynamically to the cross-sectional area of the VC at the narrowest portion of the proximal regurgitant jet. However, this simplified assumption should only hold as far as EROA is nearly circular. Asa consequence, uncertainty exists in cases in which VC width at the same time appears narrow in 4-chamber view and broad in 2-chamber view as in many cases of MR, particularly those of functional mechanism with incomplete mitral leaflet closure. Although VC width has been demonstrated to correlate with angiography and regurgitant volume and is now clinically widely used for estimating MR severity, the accuracy of VC width measurement in a 2D parasternal long-axis or apical 4-chamber view for estimation of EROA in a setting of patients with different shapes of EROA and different etiologies of MR has not been studied so far. EROA, in principle, should be directly represented by the cross-sectional area of the VC. As an important limitation, however, conventional 2D color Doppler imaging does not provide appropriate orientation of 2D scan planes to obtain a cross-sectional view of the VC area.

Regurgitant Orifice Geometry

Currently, quantification of MR based on the proximal isovelocity surface area (PISA) is one ofthe more frequently used and validated methods [18, 23, 26] To calculate an EROA by PISA, a symmetrical acceleration of flow towards the regurgitant orifice is assumed and which, in turn, creates hemispherical layers of equal velocity seen by color-flow Doppler. With 3D color Doppler, it has been proven that this geometric assumption is not always fulfilled [25] and that the measure regurgitant orifice may be underestimated.

Matsumura et al compared regurgitant orifice geometry in patients with mitral valve prolapse and patients with FMR. Patients with MVP demonstrated a spherical regurgitant orifice, whereas in those with FMR it was elliptical. Consequently, 3D color Doppler seems an appropriate technique to decide whether to use the conventional PISA method or assume a semi-elliptical shape for the mathematical calculation of regurgitant orifice area. RT3D color-flow Doppler data sets can be used for the direct quantification of MR flow volume by dealiasing of color doppler flow at the vena contracta. This RT-3D dealiasing method was feasible and appeared promising for measuring MR severity quantitatively in a spectrum of different mechanisms of mitral regurgitation and can be readily implemented in existing 3-dimensional analysis software in standard RT-3D ultrasound systems.

New generation real-time 3D TEE is a practical and feasible intraoperative technique for the rapid and accurate identification of complex MV pathology in patients referred for surgical correction of MR. RT-3D image acquisition is lesstime consuming than both traditional 3D and 2D TEE assessment of the MV and in our study was superior to 2D TEE imaging in defining specific MV pathology. Comprehensive 2D multiplanar TEE imaging remains invaluable in the Doppler assessment of MR; hence, 2D and 3D TEE imaging should be regarded as complementary, not competitive, imaging modalities.

Analysis of Mitral Prolapse

In one of the first 3DE studies, Levine et al confirmed that due to the saddle-shape of the mitralannulus, diagnosis of MV prolapse by 2D echo may be erroneous because apparent leaflet displacement toward the left atrium does not occur. This study led to a review of the diagnosis of this condition and in some laboratories its diagnosis fell by 50%. Using 3D echo, the prolapsed segment appears convex in shape when seen from the left atrium and concave when seen from the left ventricle. Using the 2D plane view (sagittal, coronal, transverse) we can choose the most appropriate plane in which to study the motion of each scallop. Sugeng et al [15] studied the use of transthoracic 3D echo in the identification of MV prolapse. The group achieved adequate MV reconstruction in 70% of cases. Probably due to its greater size, the anterior leaflet was more easily seen, both in the parasternal and apical views. The posterior leaflet was better identified from the parasternal view. Other recent studies [27, 28] compared the diagnostic efficacy of transthoracic 3DE for MV prolapse with that of transesophageal 2D echocardiography and proved both methods correlated well when image quality was adequate (89% of cases). 3D TEE (versus other echocardiographic methods) performs best when compared with anatomic examination by the surgeon during the intervention, with correct localization of the prolapsed segment in 96% of cases. Rapid, single-image acquisition with a 3D TEE probe enables the evaluation of each mitral scallop from any angle without the necessity of mental reconstruction of different echocardiographic slices. Using commercially available computer software, detailed leaflet analysis and regurgitant area measurements can be achieved and communicated to the surgeon. RT3D is a feasible, not time-consuming, non-invasive useful method in identifying the location of simple and complex lesions in patients with MV prolapse undergoing MV repair. This technique should be regarded as an important adjunct to standard 2D examination in recognizing all the components of MV leaflets and may facilitate the prediction of surgical procedures.

Implications for Heart Surgery

Mitral valve repair is the surgical treatment of choice in patients with FMR. However, it is known that up to 30% of patients sufferre current FMR during follow-up. Moreover, RT-3D echo has shown that the principal mechanism of FMR is due to adverse ventricular remodeling [29]. Prior to valve surgery a detailed study of the anatomy and function of the mitral valve should be conducted. Conventional 2D echo is severely limited in studying the 3-D structure of the MV with precision, especially in the context of FMR. RT-3D echo permits its visualization from any angle, including that of the surgeon's at the operating table. With these clear advantages, RT3D echo is becoming one of the principle tools for the surgeon both in planning and monitoring these types of surgical interventions [30, 31]. New prosthetic mitral annuloplasty devices arebeing designed in attempt to recover the originalshape of the mitral annulus and permit annular contraction and displacement as far as possible. Yamaura et al have shown that a flexible annulus provides better results than a rigid one. In this new context, RT3D echo may be used for a detailed evaluation of the geometry of the annulus and possibly help select the most appropriate prosthesis. In addition, similar studies can be conducted post-implantation to evaluate changes in annular geometry.

Due to the complex pathogenic mechanism of FMR, it is important to conduct a detailed study of mitral and ventricular geometry. To achieve reproducible measurements, it is necessary to identify the imaging plane that defines each of the cardiac structures. 2DE is limited in that all points of interest cannot be localized in one plane. This limitation is overcome with 3DE. With the development of new, user-friendly, 3D-images analysis software, the time needed to measure mitral geometry is no more than 5 minutes. The precise MR mechanism can now be elucidated using novel 3DE imaging techniques. The above-mentioned parameters that can now be measured with 3DE will surely help improve results of mitral repair. So, visualization of the annulus and mitral valves in their totality, together with analysis of subvalvular apparatus, would reveal the precise MR mechanism to the surgeon together with the degree of mitral and ventricular geometry distortion in each patient. This would facilitate individualized repair surgery planning and improve results.

Assessment of MS Using 3D Echocardiography

Rheumatic MV disease remains a major health problem, particularly in developing countries. 2D echo plays a crucial role in selecting the proper therapeutic strategy in patients with MS.1 Apart from estimation of the trans-mitral pressure gradient; 2D echo can calculate MVA by planimetry and pressure half-time. The diagnosis and determination of the severity of mitral stenosis is based on 2D echo and Doppler techniques. The determination of valvular area with Doppler (pressure half-time or continuity method or proximal convergence flow) is the most commonly used technique. However, it is accepted that these methods are influenced by hemodynamicstatus (heart rate, cardiac rhythm, cardiac output), the compliance of the ventricle, and the presence of other associated valvular lesions. Planimetered mitral area methods are not affectedby hemodynamic changes so they are widely used today. However, planimetry requires the correct orientation of the plane to obtain the smallest area traced from the leaflets' free edge, and oblique slices can overestimate mitral area. RT3D echo is a rapid, precise technique for determiningthe valvular orifice area, as it facilitates the orientation of any slice plane to locate the minimal MV area. Thus, it eliminates one of the principle limitations of 2D echo in determining mitral valve area by planimetry. Several studies have compared 3D echo with traditional methods of calculating MV area.39-41 The mitral area measured using RT3D echo planimetry correlates better with Gorlin's formula than do traditional 2D echocardiographic methods. Moreover, with RT3DE there is less inter- and intra-observer variation when calculating mitral valve area. Also, 2DE is essential in the selection of patients for percutaneous mitral valvuloplasty. Among all available MV scoring systems, Wilkins score is the most commonly used. This score evaluates MV thickness, mobility (figure 14), leaflet calcification (figure

15), and the degree of subvalvular apparatus thickening. A favorable Wilkins score (<8 points) is highly predictive of a good outcome after percutaneous mitral valvuloplasty. More recently, it has been shown that other factors, such as commissural fusion and calcification, are also strong predictors of outcomes after percutaneous mitral valvuloplasty [32].

The introduction of RT3D echo and advances in analysis software have improved MVorientation and evaluation.11 Several studies have reported improved accuracy and superiority of RT3D echo over 2D echo for MVA estimation. RT3D echo allows a unique ''en face'' view and morphologic analysis ofthe entire MV apparatus, including the MV annulus, the subvalvular apparatus, and its anatomic relation to other nearby structures. Recently, 3D echo has been introduced and theoretically offersadvantages for quantification, by allowing generation of a series of equidistant parallel cross sectionsthrough the mitral valve apparatus). Thus the smallest orifice area can be identified, and planimetry performed. No significant differences were found between MVA derived by 3D echo and values obtained by Doppler PHT methods.

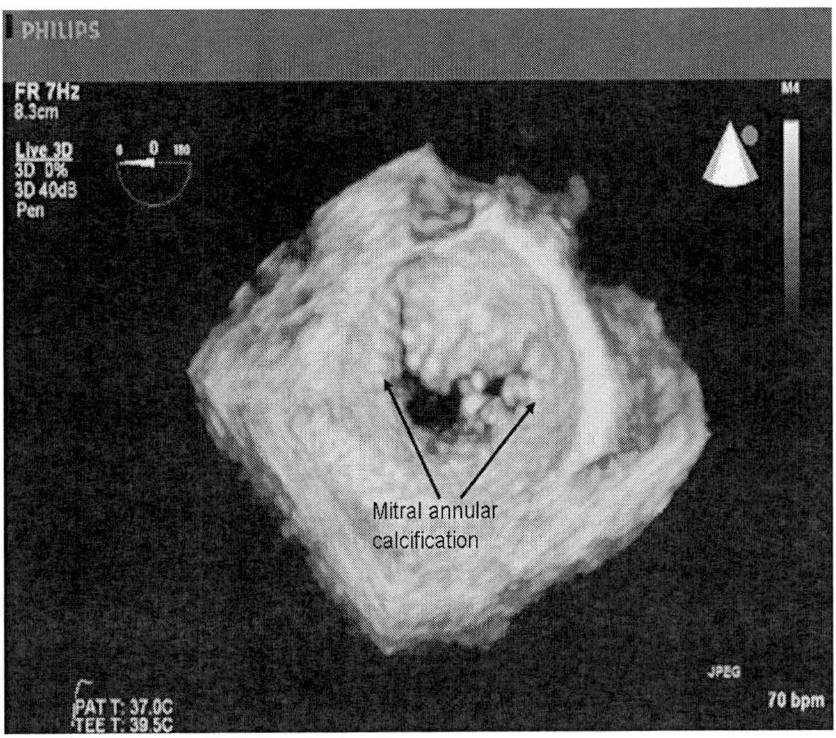

Figure 15. restricted posterior leaflet movement due to leaflet calcification.

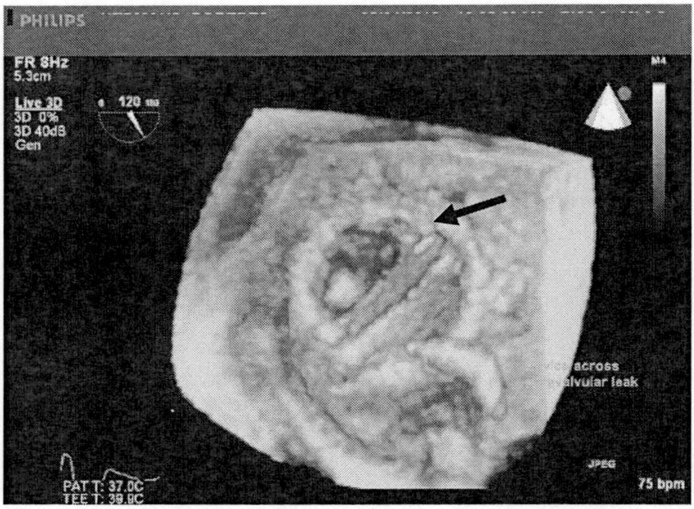

Figure 16. Dehiscence of mitral prosthesis (arrow).

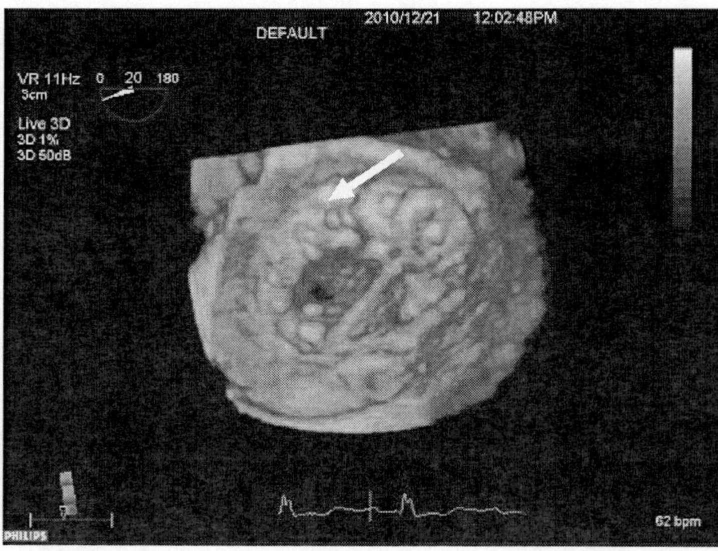

Figure 17. Percutaneous closure of mitral paravalvular leak with Amplatzer PDA occluder (arrow).

The greatest advantage of acquiring a 3D echo image data set is that cross-sectional images of a structurecan be generated in any plane desired independently from orientations dictated by the acoustic windows. Electronic parallel slicing allows the selection of parallel cut planes in a way similar to that of computed tomography or magnetic resonance imaging to select the cut plane with the smallest orifice area. 3D echo thus allows more accurate measurement of the orifice areain patients with MS.

LIMITATIONS OF THE CURRENT 3D TEE FOR MV EVALUATION

The main limitations of the current systems are the small field of view in real-time modes and the relatively slow frame rate, equivalent to only 20 to 30 frames/s. This permits the capture of only 5 to 7 frames on some loops. An additional shortcoming of the present technology is the lack of color Doppler in the real-time formats. Color Doppler can be acquired only in the large-sector format or in the simultaneous biplane format. There is also room for improvement of the spatial resolution of the current systems. Very fine structures such as chordate tendineae are not well visualized. The details of the ventricular surfaceof the mitral valve are also more difficult to discern and can present artifacts, giving the appearance of cobblestones. Table 7 illustrates some of the strengths and weaknesses of 3D Echocardiography as compared to 2D.

FUTURE PROSPECTIVE

Ongoing developments in 3D echocardiography include technological innovations and expandingclinical applications. Automated surface extraction and quantification, single-heartbeat full-volumeacquisition, transesophageal RT-3D imaging, the ability to navigate within the 3D volume, andstereoscopic visualization of 3D images are some of the technological advances that can be expectedover the next several years. These will further enhance the quality and clinical applicationsof 3D echocardiography. In addition, standardized and focused 3D protocols will be developedand refined to optimize clinical application of this technique. Tagging and/or tracking the LV surface in real time may provide new approaches to quantifying myocardial mechanics, such as regional shape and strain. This approach has great potential and will complement and likely compare favorably withthe quantitative ability of cardiac MRI. The superior temporal resolution of RT-3D echocardiography provides a clear view of distinct flail segments of the MV, which will be a fertile area for clinical research that will likely show the superiority of this new method in the patient selection for mitral valve repair procedures. Additionally, the use of this technology to guide interventional procedures like MV balloon valvuloplasties and E-valve clip repairs could have a great potential. The detailed structural and functional analysis of the mitral annulus now possible with 3D TEE will facilitate investigations directed at differentiating structural from FMR.

Implications of RT-3D Echocardiogram in Percutaneous Treatment of Mitral Disease

The application of echocardiography in the cardiac catheterization laboratory has facilitated certain interventions and has allowed the timely detection of procedural complications. In recent years we have witnessed the incorporation of transesophageal and intra-cardiac 2D echo in the catheterization laboratory for guidance of percutaneous procedures. Given the additional advantages of RT3D echo over existing echocardiographic modalities, the time is right for its use in the guidance of similar procedures. As mentioned earlier, RT3D echo can also be particularly useful in determining mitral valve area in patients with MS and it could reliably be applied in percutaneous mitral valvuloplasty procedures. This is especially interesting if we consider how imprecise immediate, conventional non-invasive post-procedural techniques are. Similarly, RT3D echo could be of use in guiding the inter-atrial wall puncture needed in mitral device implantation. 3D visualization of the entire mitral annulus prosthesis in patients with periprosthetic leaks (figure 16) obviates the mental reconstruction necessary to localize their origin and, consequently, improves diagnostic precision. Although there is minimal scientific evidence to support it, the application of RT-3D echo may provide great advantage in the guidance of percutaneous closure procedures for periprosthetic leaks [33] (figure 17). Moreover, it will be able to guide MV procedures such as the Alfieri percutaneous repair technique or mitral annuloplasty ring implantation via the coronary sinus [34].

REFERENCES

[1] Gutiérrez-Chico J.L., ZamoranoGómez J.L., Rodrigo-López J.L., et al: Accuracy of real-time 3-dimensional echocardiography in the assessment Is transesophageal echocardiography still mandatory? *Am Heart J* 2008; 155:694-698.

[2] Textbook of Clinical Echocardiography, 4th Edition, *Catherine M.* Otto, MD.

[3] Levine R.A., Schwammenthal E.: Ischemic mitral regurgitation *Circulation* 2005; 112:745-758.

[4] Monin J.L., Dehant P., Roiron C., et al: Functional assessment. *J Am Coll Cardiol* 2005; 46:302-309.

[5] Grigioni F., Enriquez-Sarano M., Zehr K.J., et al: Ischemic mitral regurgitation *Circulation* 2001; 103:1759-1764.

[6] Kim Y.J., Jones M., Greenberg N.L., et al: Evaluation. *J Am Soc Echocardiogr* 2007; 20:1086-1092.

[7] Zoghbi W.A., Enriquez-Sarano M., Foster E., et al: Recommendations for evaluation of the severity of native valvular regurgitation with two-dimensional and Doppler echocardiography. *J Am Soc* Echocardiogr 2003; 16:777-802.

[8] Bonow R.O., Carabello B.A., Chatterjee K., et al: ACC/AHA 2006 guidelines *J Am CollCardiol* 2006; 48:e1-e148.

[9] Robert B.J., Grayburn P.A.: Color flow imaging of the vena contracta in mitral regurgitation J Am Soc Echocardiogr 2003; 16:1002-1006.

[10] Summa Matsumura Y., Fukuda S., Tran H., et al: Geometry of the proximal isovelocity surface area *Am Heart J* 2008; 155:231-238.

[11] Henry W.L., Griffith J.M., Michaelis L.L., et al: Measurement of mitral orifice area in patients with mitral valve *Circulation* 1975; 51:827-831.

[12] Hatle L., Angelsen B., Tromsdal A.: Noninvasive assessment *Circulation* 1979; 60:1096-1104.

[13] Baumgartner H., Hung J., Bermejo J., et al: Echocardiographic assessment *J Am Soc Echocardiogr* 2009; 22:1-23.

[14] Carabello B.A.: Modern management. *Circulation* 2005; 112:432-437.

[15] Sugeng L, Shernan SK, Salgo IS, et al. Live 3-dimensional transesophageal echocardiography: initial experience using the fully sampled matrix array probe. *J Am CollCardiol* 2008;52:446 –9.

[16] A. Bhan, S Kapetanakis, M. J. Monaghan. Three-dimensional echocardiography. *Heart* 2010;96:153–163.

[17] Judy Hung, MD, Roberto Lang, MD, Frank Flachskampf, MD Et al.3D Echocardiography: A Review of the Current Status and Future Directions.*J Am Soc Echocardiogr* 2007;20:213-233.

[18] Anne-Sophie Beraud, MD, IngelaSchnittger, MD, D. Craig Miller, MD Etal. Multiplanar Reconstruction of Three-Dimensional Transthoracic Echocardiography Improves the Presurgical Assessment of Mitral Prolapse.*J Am Soc Echocardiogr* 2009;22:907-13.

[19] Annette Vegas, MD, FRCPC, and MassimilianoMeineri, MD. Three-Dimensional Transesophageal Echocardiography Is a Major Advance for Intraoperative Clinical Management of Patients *Undergoing Cardiac Surgery: A Core Review.* (AnesthAnalg 2010;110:1548 –73).

[20] Gloria Tamborini*, Manuela Muratori, Anna Maltagliati. Pre-operative transthoracic real-time three-dimensional echocardiography in patients undergoing mitral valve repair: accuracy in cases with simple vs. complex prolapse lesions. *European Journal of Echocardiography* (2010) 11, 778–785.

[21] Jorge Solis,a Marta Sitges,b Robert A. Levine,a and Judy Hunga Et al. Three-Dimensional Echocardiography. New Possibilities in Mitral Valve Assessment. *Rev EspCardiol*. 2009;62 (2):188-98.

[22] S.A. Kleijn, O. Kamp. Clinical application of three-dimensional echocardiography: past, present and future. *Neth HeartJ* 2009;17:18-24.).

[23] Ernesto E. Salcedo, MD, Robert A. Quaife, MD Et al. A Framework for Systematic Characterization of the Mitral Valve by Real-Time Three-Dimensional Transesophageal Echocardiography. *J Am Soc Echo cardiogry* 2009;22:1087-99.

[24] Hyun Suk Yang, MD, PhD, Ramesh C. Bansal, MD, FASE, Et al. Practical Guide for Three-Dimensional Transthoracic Echocardiography Using a Fully Sampled Matrix Array Transducer. *J Am Soc of Echo cardiography,* September 2008 Volume 21 Number 9.

[25] Philipp Kahlert, MD, Björn Plicht, MD, Ingmar M. Schenk, MD Et al. Direct Assessment of Size and Shape of Noncircular Vena Contracta Area in Functional Versus Organic Mitral Regurgitation Using Real-Time Three-Dimensional *Echocardiography J Am Soc of Echo cardiography* 21, 8 August 2008.

[26] BjörnPlicht, MD, Philipp Kahlert, MD, RannyGoldwasser Et al. Direct Quantification of Mitral Regurgitant Flow Volume by Real-Time Three-Dimensional Echocardiography Using Dealiasing of Color Doppler

Flow at the Vena Contracta *J Am Soc Echocardiogr* 2008;21:1337-1346.

[27] Mauro Pepi, MD, Gloria Tamborini, MD, Anna Maltagliati, MD et al Head-to-Head Comparison of Two- and Three-Dimensional Transthoracic and Transesophageal Echocardiography in the Localization of Mitral Valve Prolapse *J Am CollCardiol* 2006;48:2524 – 30.

[28] Rajan Sharma, MD, MRCP, Jon Mann, MRCP, Linda Drummond, MSC Et al The Evaluation of Real-time 3-Dimensional Transthoracic Echo cardiography for the Preoperative Functional Assessment of Patients with Mitral Valve Prolapse: A Comparison with 2-Dimensional Transesophageal Echocardiography. *J Am Soc Echocardiogr* 2007;20:934-940.).

[29] Jeffrey J. Silbiger, MD, FASE, Mechanistic Insights into Ischemic Mitral Regurgitation: Echocardiographic and Surgical Implications. *J Am Soc Echocardiogr* 2011.

[30] Jeng Wei, Ming C. Hsiung, Shen Kou Tsai Et al. The routine use of live three-dimensional transesophageal echocardiography in mitral valve surgery: clinical experience. *European Journal of Echocardiography* (2010) 11, 14–18.

[31] Jasmine Grewal, MD, Sunil Mankad, MD, William K. Freeman, MD, Et al Real-Time Three-Dimensional Transesophageal Echocardiography in the Intraoperative Assessment of Mitral Valve Disease (*J Am Soc Echocardiogr* 2009;22:34-41).

[32] JorinaLangerveld, MD, Gabriel Valocik, MD, H. W. ThijsPlokker, MD, PhD Et al. Additional Value of Three-dimensional Transesophageal Echocardiography for Patients with Mitral Valve Stenosis Undergoing Balloon Valvuloplasty (*J Am Soc Echocardiogr* 2003;16:841-9.).

[33] ItzhakKronzon, MD,*LissaSugeng, MD,† Gila Perk, MD Et al Real-Time 3-Dimensional Transesophageal Echocardiography in the Evaluation of Post-Operative Mitral Annuloplasty Ring and Prosthetic Valve Dehiscence. *J Am CollCardiol* 2009;53:1543–7.

[34] Simon Biner, MD, Gila Perk, MD, FASE, SaibalKar, MD. Et al. Utility of Combined Two-Dimensional and Three-Dimensional Transesophageal Imaging for Catheter-Based Mitral Valve Clip Repair of Mitral Regurgitation. (*J Am Soc Echocardiogr* 2011;24:611-7.).

In: Mitral Valve Disease
Editor: Richard R. Heuser
ISBN: 978-1-61942-309-1

Chapter 5

CT AND MRI EVALUATION OF MITRAL VALVE DISEASES

Zhi-gang Yang and Wen Deng
Department of Radiology, West China Hospital, Sichuan University, Chengdu, Sichuan, China

Mitral valve diseases result in structural and functional changes in the mitral complex caused by congenital anomalies or acquired pathogenic factors. The symptoms of mitral valve disease are mitral stenosis or mitral regurgitation. There are a few cases of congenital mitral lesions, and acquired mitral lesions are the most common in underdeveloped countries, particularly in the form of rheumatic mitral valve disease, whereas the most common mitral valve disease in developed countries is mitral valve prolapse [1-4]. The earliest diagnostic techniques for mitral lesions were cardioangiography and heart catheterization, but traumatic examinations have gradually been replaced by the ultrasonic cardiogram [2]. Twenty years ago, cardiovascular magnetic resonance (CMR) emerged as the gold standard for assessing heart function. In some developed countries, CMR is also an important supplementary measure for diagnosing and grading mitral lesions [5]. Ultrasonic cardiogram and CMR have their respective advantages and limitations for diagnosing mitral lesions. For example, the ultrasonic cardiogram shows poor repetition, whereas CMR is expensive. In recent years, with the rapid growth of imaging technology, computed tomography (CT) has been used to observe the shape and function of the mitral valve [6]. Currently, CT is not applied widely to clinically diagnose valvular heart disease, and few studies have been conducted except for a few cases of mitral lesions. In this chapter, imaging evaluation of mitral valve disease and related cardiac function changes were reviewed.

I. Causes and Pathological Characteristics of Mitral Lesions

Mitral valve diseases can be divided into mitral stenosis, mitral regurgitation, and mitral stenosis accompanied by regurgitation.

In mitral stenosis, it is difficult for the blood to flow into the left ventricle during the left ventricle l diastole phase as a result of changes in the shape and function of the mitral complex. In 1954, Wood first described the clinical characteristics of mitral stenosis [7]. The most common cause of mitral stenosis is rheumatic fever, which has high prevalence worldwide. In different regions, this disease may have different incidence rates. Before the 1960s, both developed and underdeveloped countries had nearly the same incidence of rheumatic fever, but currently, the highest incidence is seen in the Middle East and Africa. In the past 30–40 years, the incidence of rheumatic fever has decreased remarkably in developed countries [1, 2, 8]. For example, in the US, the incidence of rheumatic fever among pre-school children is 0.6/1000 persons; in Asia, the number is 0.4–21.0/1000 persons; and in China, it has been controlled at <1/1000 in the past 30 years [3].

In mitral regurgitation, the blood from the left ventricle flows into the left atrium through an incompletely closed cardiac valve orifice during the left ventricular sistole phase as a result of changes in the shape and function of the mitral complex. The cause of mitral regurgitation is most frequently mitral valve prolapse [4], whereas the most common cause in China still remains rheumatic fever.

In addition, the most common causes for mitral valve disease include mitral degeneration, ischemic mitral valve disease, and congenital heart disease. The pathological features of the common causes for mitral lesions are as follows:

1. Rheumatic Mitral Valve Disease

Rheumatic fever is an autoimmune disease caused by a *Streptococcus* pharyngeal infection and the fever associated with the disease affects mitral function. When Group A β-*Streptococcus hemolyticus* invades the human body through the pharynx, it stimulates the production of antibodies, which attack the *Streptococcus* and act on the connective tissues of the mitral valve to cause monocytic and serous effusion, lesions, and necrosis. The inflammatory exudates are absorbed by hyperplasia-triggered macrophages to form Aschoff knur, and finally they contain fibroblast cells and collagenous fibers, which form scars [1, 9]. When rheumatic fever strikes repeatedly, these pathological processes can be repeated in the mitral valve, aggravating degenerative swelling and scar formation and causing changes to mitral valve structure and function.

2. Mitral Valve Prolapse

Mitral valve prolapse means that the mitral valve cusp proceeds in waves toward the left atrium during the contraction phase of the heart. A 1958 study mentioned a clicking sound in the middle and late contraction phases and the authors stated that this originated from outside the heart [10]. However, 5 years later, Barlow et al. demonstrated using left ventriculography that the sound was caused by mitral valve prolapse [11]. Several years later, Criley et al. summarized the clinical expression by conducting angiography and grading the pathology [12]. General mitral valve prolapse includes primary mitral valve prolapse and secondary mitral valve prolapse (caused by rheumatic fever, coronary heart disease, or hypertrophic cardiomyopathy). Primary mitral valve prolapse reveals mucoid degeneration as the pathology. During slight degeneration, the mitral valve cusp gets longer and drops slightly into the left ventricle, without clinical symptoms, whereas after significant degeneration, the valve becomes thicker, the cusp gets longer, and the tendinous cord becomes extended or even ruptures, with the clinical expression of serious mitral regurgitation [1, 4].

3. Degeneration among the Elderly and Calcification of the Mitral Annulus

In the early stage after birth, the mitral valve is translucent. However, the mitral valve gradually develops fibrosis and fat sediment with age and finally the nodule thickens and a valve annulus lesion calcifies, which is closely related with high blood pressure and high blood fat. Mitral stenosis occurs when calcification of the valve annulus reaches a particular stage, and mitral regurgitation occurs with extreme calcification of the valve annulus. Other than age, calcification of the valve annulus is caused by Marfan syndrome, mitral valve prolapse, Hurler syndrome, and secondary hyperparathyroidism among patients with kidney failure.

4. Ischemic Mitral Valve Disease and Papillary Muscle Dysfunction

The mitral front-valve papillary muscles supply blood through the ramus anterior descendens and the diagonal branch of the obtuse marginal branch of the left circumflex artery, whereas the back-valve papillary muscles are supplied by the posterior descending branch. Papillary muscle infarcts occur when coronary heart disease involves these blood vessels, and the relationship between the papillary muscles and the tendinous cord changes, which results in mitral regurgitation. Additionally, shock, severe anemia, heart tumors, and amyloidosis also cause papillary muscle dysfunction.

II. Noninvasive Mitral Diagnostics

1. Three-position Cardiac X-ray Radiography

Before the emergence of ultrasonic imaging, the mitral valve could not be observed non-invasively, except through indirect signs to identify its basic shape and function. The three-position heart diagnosis is the oldest measure to diagnose mitral valve lesions. Using this technique, we can identify whether the heart ventricle boundaries have enlarged or not, and detect the expression of the porta pulmonis and blood distribution inside the lung. Therefore, functional changes in the mitral valve can be indirectly ascertained. When the mitral valve has obvious calcification, mitral valve changes can be directly visualized on an X-ray plan drawing. However, it is still difficult to provide an accurate diagnosis for a mitral valve lesion. Additionally, the radiation used during the test limits its clinical application. However, the three-position heart diagnostic was a typical test that doctors used to diagnose mitral valve diseases.

2. Echocardiogram

In 1942, an Austrian named Dussik began to use a Model A ultrasonic device to detect the brain, which ushered in ultrasonic imaging. In the 1950s and 1960s, Model M, Model B, and Doppler ultrasonic wave imaging machines were then introduced and applied clinically. In 1954, Edler et al. used ultrasonic waves to evaluate heart structure and movement, leading to the debut of the ultrasonic cardiogram for clinical use [13]. In the 1970s, Doppler ultrasonic waves were applied to ultrasonic cardiograms, and heart blood kinetic parameters were measured noninvasively. Shape and functional changes in the mitral valve and the valve passage area can be observed and assessed, and the transvalvular pressure gradient, regurgitant volume, and regurgitant signal range can be calculated using an ultrasonic cardiogram. Thus, the ultrasonic cardiogram became the classic gold standard for diagnosing mitral valve lesions [2]. The ultrasonic cardiogram is noninvasive and has become the most economical and simplest measure to assess the mitral valve, which has made it the first-choice clinically. The ultrasonic cardiogram is also the most flexible imaging test but creates high demands on the operational skills and clinical experience of the tester The limitation of this method is that different testers may collect different clinical information. In the past 30 years, three-dimensional ultrasonic cardiograms have been developed and have become the best technology for observing mitral valve lesions after 2000, as they offer more accurate images and functional parameters of mitral valve lesions and may possibly overcome the over dependence of ultrasonic cardiograms on the tester [14-16].

3. Computed Tomography (CT)

When CT emerged more than 40 years ago, it could not be applied to assess the heart. Only with the emergence of electron beam CT (EBCT), multi-row detector CT (MDCT), and dual-source CT (DSCT) has coronary angio graphy matured and become popular. EBCT is a CT device that is completely different from normal CT designs, as it uses an electron gun with extremely high resolution (resolution as high as 100 ms), which is suitable for heart scanning. But EBCT does not collect isotropic voxel data, so it cannot be used for restructuring complicated shapes, and its cost is high. EBCT also cannot be used to check other parts of the body, so it has usability drawbacks. Two major technical advances have been made in the development of heart CT, i.e., improvements in gantry rotation speed and the use of multi-row detectors. The MDCT has wider coverage and the ability to collect multiple slices of imaging data with one rotation of the X-ray tube, and four-slice CT machines emerged based on this capability. By 1998, four-slice MDCT of which scanning thickness is about 1.25–1.5 mm had emerged, and its collecting speed was slow (approximately 0.5–0.8 s/cycle, and the scanning coverage remained small (dozens of cms), and therefore, MDCT could not ideally display the heart and coronary artery. The development of a 16-slice MDCT realized isotropic voxel collection, which made reconstructing an image real and laid the foundation for various complicated reconstruction technologies. But, the 16-slice MDCT's detector width was still narrow, so scanning durations were long, and the resolution was still insufficient to clearly display the heart and coronary arteries. The 64-slice MDCT, produced at the end of 2003, collects 64 slices images at once, has scanning speeds of 0.33–0.35 s/cycle, and provides improved information-collecting temporal resolution, allowing for coronary artery testing and heart imaging. But, the wider detector also resulted in larger cone-shaped harness artifacts, more complicated calibration algorithms, and the necessity for super-large computers to analyze the huge volumes of scanning data. In 2005, DSCT was first introduced, which is a new-concept machine that changed the basic structures of traditional CT machines. These instruments used double spherical tubes and double detectors, combined the fly focus technology, and improved heart CT imaging temporal resolution to 83 ms, omitted heart rate and heart rhythm factors, resulting in high-quality coronary artery imaging. Furthermore, the DSCT equipment has also made remarkable progress in reducing the radiation dose.

Many studies have applied EBCT, MDCT, and DSCT to valvular heart diseases. MDCT and DSCT normally have cine CT and volume-phase display patterns, and the collected data can be analyzed with many types of software and treated with maximum intensity projection, multiplanar reconstruction, and a volume rendering technique to clearly show the anatomy of the heart ventricles, accurately locate the heart valves, measure blood dynamic parameters at different timed phases of the heart cycle, and offer valuable clinical information. Thus, MDCT and DSCT are very useful supplementary imaging tests to clinically diagnose valvular heart disease [17]. Few heart CT studies have been conducted for mitral valve lesions, but based on the current clinical applications of CT to valvular heart diseases, CT can accurately assess the severity of mitral valve lesions and detect lesion-led functional changes in the heart [6,18-24]. Today, CT has been applied to the basic study of mitral valve lesions. Its disadvantages are its high cost and high radiation dose.

4. Magnetic Resonance Imaging (MRI)

MRI was first used for medical diagnosis in the 1970s, and cardiovascular magnetic resonance (CMR) for valvular heart disease diagnosis has about a 20 year history, with the major technologies of steady-state free precession cine, gradient echo cine, phase contrast, turbo-spin echo (T1, T2, with or without fat saturation), and segmented inversion recovery gradient echo. With these technologies, CMR displays better mitral valve location and anatomy than that displayed by an ultrasonic cardiogram and is the gold standard for heart function assessment [5,25-27]. Currently, CMR is a major supplementary test for valvular heart disease diagnoses, but is not clinically popular, which may be due to factors such as high cost and long imaging time [5]. Table 1 shows the advantages and disadvantages of the various heart testing methods described.

III. Normal Mitral Valve Imaging Expression

The mitral valve is located at the left atrium and is composed of two valves; a front valve that extends from the noncoronary sinus of the aortic valve, which is longer, and a back valve that is located on the back outside of the valve annulus, which is wider. The two valve edges are connected through the tendinous cord and the papillary muscles of the left ventricle. The mitral valve, together with the mitral valve annulus, tendinous cord, and papillary muscles is called the mitral valve complex. Under normal conditions, the mitral valve complex is complete and coordinated in movement, as the mitral valve annulus and valve orifice open and change regularly with movement of the mitral valve complex.

Table 1. Advantages and Disadvantages of Various Testing Methods

Testing method	Advantages	Disadvantages
Three-position cardiac X-ray radiography	Easy operation Low cost	Indirect diagnosis of mitral valve lesions Radiation
Echocardiogram	Direct display of the mitral valve shape Easy operation Low cost No radiation Standard references for mitral valve lesions No contrast agents No post-processing reconstruction after imaging acqusition	Poor repeatability Limited by acoustic windows for the pictures
CT	Direct display of the mitral valve anatomy Short scanning time High time and space resolution Good repetition Sensitive to calcified lesions	Radiation High cost Need contrast agents Long time for post-processing reconstruction Inaccurate measuring of mitral valve-related blood flow dynamic parameters
MRI	Direct display of the mitral valve anatomy Accurate measuring of cardiac functional parameters Good repetition Accurate measuring of mitral valve-related blood flow dynamic parameters No radiation No contrast agents No post-processing reconstruction after imaging acqusition	High cost Long time of imaging acquisition Unsuitability for patients with metal articles in their bodies and claustrophobics

Improved CT and MRI technologies have allowed the mitral valve to be observed, and on the heart long-axis plan the mitral valves are two connected or unconnected thin-thread structures extending toward the heart ventricles, whereas on the heart short-axis plan, the soft tissues are in fish-mouth shapes or lines in the left heart ventricle.

Using cine CT and many post-processing software applications, CT and MRI can display the shapes and changes in the mitral valve during the different cardiac cycles and on different sections. The cardiac cycles can be divided into an isovolumic contraction period, a rapid ejection period, a slow ejection period, an isovolumic relaxation period, a rapid flow period, a reduced filling period, and an atrial systole period. The reconstruction time phases on CT are 0%, 10%, 20%, 30%, 40%, 50%, 60%, 70%, 80% and 90%, basically corresponding to the cardiac cycle periods [28]. The mitral valve is closed in arch-like shape (section and heart long-axis plan) or thread-like shape (heart short-axis plan) on the reconstructed time phases of 0%, 10%, 20%, 30%, and 40% and is opened on the time phases of 50%, 60%, 70%, 80%, and 90%, in the sluice type (section and heart long-axis plan) or fish-mouth (heart short-axis plan) shape. The movements of the normal mitral valve during the cardiac periods are such that the mitral annular area (MAA) is at a minimum at the 0% time phase and increases along with the time phase of cardiac cycle movement. When the time phase is 80%, the MAA will be at a maximum. The diameter of the mitral annulus decreases between 80% and 0%, and rises stably between 0% and 50%, and then stay almost still between 50% and 80%. The mitral valve area (MVA) and diameter increases between 30% and 40%, and is maximum at 90% but decreases sharply between 90% and 0% and becomes zero at systole phases. The opening angle of the anterior valve is at a minimum at 30% and a maximum at the 60% time phase with the anterior valve change range larger than that of the posterior valve. The opening angle of the posterior valve is at a minimum at 30% and a maximum at the 90% time phase.

IV. Mitral Valve Disease and Heart Functional Changes on Imaging

1. Mitral Stenosis

At the early stage of mitral stenosis, due to various reasons, the left ventricle develops a filling disorder during diastole, whereas the left atrium develops compensatory hypertrophy to increase left atrial pressure, making blood pass rapidly through the narrow space and causing torrential flow and shake, which is clinically expressed as a rumbling noise at the apex area of the heart during diastole. Adhesive connections can be visualized at the boundary of the anterior and posterior valves on CT. The valves are thickened, sometimes calcified (Figure 1), with reduced MVA (Figure 2), shortened tendon adhesions, thickened papillary muscles and decreased left ventricular end diastolic volume (LVEDV).

If allowed to progress, the left atrium develops broken compensation, and blood flow backs up, causing a pulmonary vein blood backflow obstruction, pulmonary congestion, edema and even diapedetic hemorrhage, with clinical dyspnea, cyanopathy, cough, and other left atrium failure symptoms. On CT, mitral stenoses produce left atrial dilatation, pulmonary vein dilation, pulmonary vein disorder, and occasionally left atrial mural thrombi, i.e., contrast-agent filling defects.

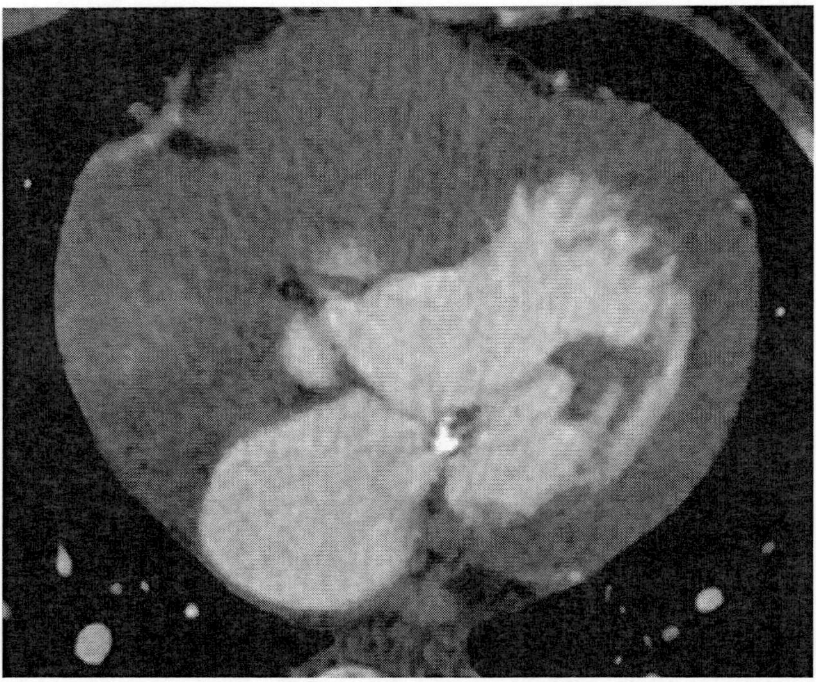

Figure 1. This image shows mitral leaflet calcification of a 64-year old man with rheumatic heart disease on the axial plane.

During the late stages of the disease, the pulmonary congestion causes pulmonary artery spasms, which increase pulmonary arterial pressure, causing the right ventricle to develop decompensation dilation from compensatory hypertrophy, incomplete closure of the tricuspid valve, and finally resulting in right heart failure featured by right ventricular and circulatory congestion. The symptoms are an increase in right ventricular end systolic volume (RVESV); a decrease in right ventricular stroke volume (RVSV), the right ventricular ejection fraction (RVEF), and right ventricular end diastolic volume (RVEDV); and a right ventricular wall mass (RV-mass) increase or decrease. Some patients develop thoracic pericardial effusion, and slight shrinking of the left ventricle.

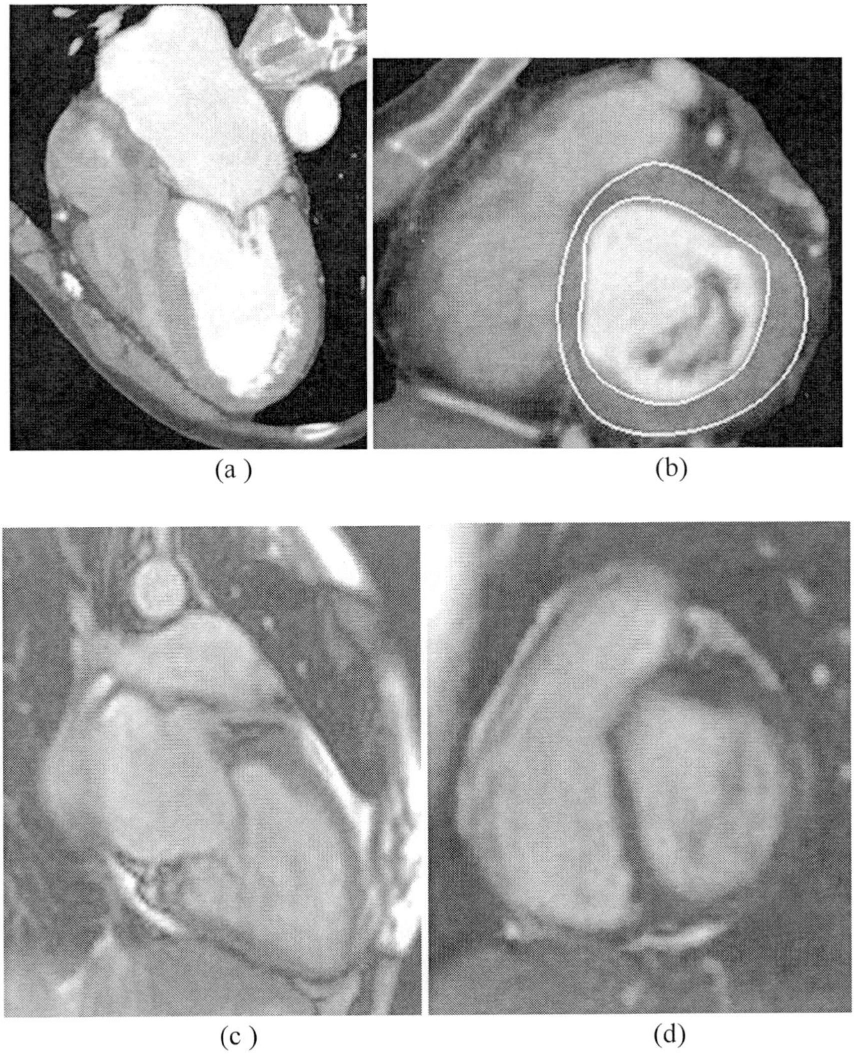

Figure 2. This series of image shows CT (a, b) and MRI (c, d) manifestations of a 17-year old girl with severe rheumatic mitral stenosis. Mitral leaflets hardly opened during diastole on the long-axis plane (a, c). The mitral valve area (MVA) was quite narrow, shaped like crescent on the short-axis plane during the whole diastole.

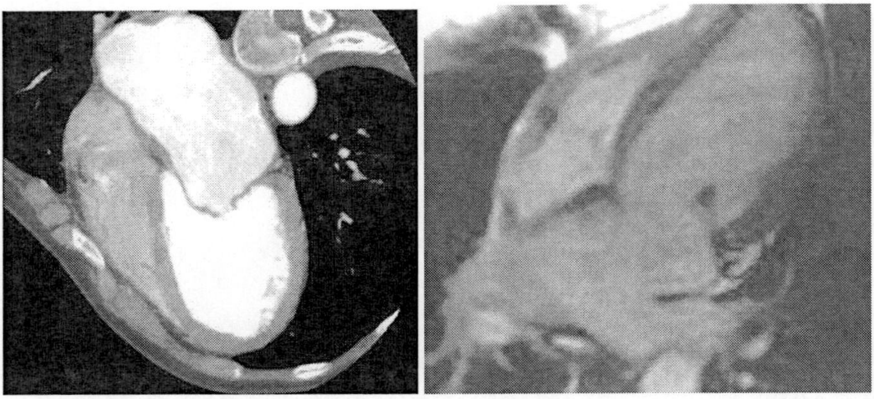

(a) (b)

Figure 3. This series of image shows CT (a) and MRI (b) manifestation of a 31-year old woman with mitral regurgitation. Mitral leaflets couldn't close completely during systole on the long-axis plane. Left atrial enlargement is another obvious manifestation.

The degree of mitral stenosis should be assessed by MVA measured by ultrasonic cardiogram. Studies have demonstrated that 64-MDCT can accurately and dynamically display a normal mitral valve and measure relevant mitral valve and heart function parameters, indicating that it is feasible to use CT to diagnose mitral stenosis. [29, 30]

For MRI, a mitral valve with stenosis is limited and has the symptoms of a small openness of a cine MRI displayed valve, an abnormal shape, and a connected valve relationship (Figure 2), with football and ejection symptoms, indicating signal loss due to the rapid blood flow signal through the mitral stenosis. Then, the blood arrives at the left ventricle directional low-bundle signal area of the mitral valve during the heart diastole phase. The scope and area percentage of the left ventricle have a good relationship with mitral stenosis, and mitral stenosis should be assessed in a semi-quantitative way. MRI also is also capable of directly displaying the valve's shape, size, thickness, excrescence, and activity. The thickness and size of the valve should be measured using the left ventricle long-axis sequence perpendicular to the ventricular septum and parallel to the interval. The thickness and movement of the valve can be displayed with bright cine MRI in terms of contraction period and the shape of the valve during diastole. Similar to CT, cine MRI perpendicular to the ventricular septum and parallel to the interval can be used to directly measure the diameter of the valve annulus during contraction and relaxation. In addition, MRI is also useful for measuring mean flow velocity, maximum blood flow velocity, forward blood flow, and reverse blood flow The left atrial and left ventricular transvalvular pressure gradient should be calculated according to the simplified Bernoulli equation to estimate and measure the degree of mitral valve stenosis. While displaying the enlarged left atrium, MRI can detect a left atrial thrombus. A left atrial thrombus often originates from the left atrium or the left atrial lateral wall. Spin-echo may have different signals according to different times of thrombus formation, and a T2WI thrombus has a relatively low range of signals. No apparent enhancement of the thrombus will be seen if gadolinium diethylenetriamine pentaacetic acid-enhanced scanning is applied. Heart long and short axis section MRI images display enlargement of the right ventricle and the thickness of the locular wall.

2. Mitral Regurgitation

In the early stage of mitral valve regurgitation, blood regurgitates into the left atrium through the valve orifice during contraction of the left ventricle to enlarge the left atrium, producing a blood vortex and blowing noise at the apex area of the heart during holosystole. Then, the left ventricle, due to excessive filling at diastole, develops compensatory hypertrophy, with CT revealing valve thickening, fibrosis, and calcification. At 0%–40% time phases, the mitral valve cannot close, the left atrium and ventricle become enlarged (Figure 3), and the LVEDV is augmented.

In the middle stage of the disease, the left atrium and ventricle successively enter a decompensatory stage, resulting in pulmonary congestion. CT shows pulmonary vein dilation, pulmonary vein disorder, and a decrease in LVEDV. Notably, patients with chronic mitral valve regurgitation will experience a long duration from the early-stage CT symptoms to the middle stage CT symptoms compared with patients who have acute mitral valve regurgitation and mitral stenosis.

In the end stage of the disease, patients gradually develop right heart failure and systemic congestion due to pulmonary hypertension. Furthermore, besides the left ventricular changes, CT shows the same findings as with the end-stage mitral stenosis, including right atrial and right ventricular enlargement, increased RVESV, decreased RVSV and RVEF, and RVEDV and RV-mass augmentation or shrinking.

The severity of mitral valve regurgitation is graded clinically mainly using the ultrasonic cardiogram. Recently, comparative studies have been conducted about the severity of simple mitral valve regurgitation and heart function parameters in terms of 64-MDCT, MRI, and transthoracic echocardiography (TTE). According to reports, the 64-MDCT results are consistent with those of TTE when the severity of mitral valve regurgitation and its measured heart functional parameters are the same statistically with the results of MRI [29-32].

On cine MRI, blood regurgitation of the mitral valve is expressed as a blood signal flowing into the left atrium through the mitral valve during contraction that is lost due to regurgitation and flow into the bundle low-signal area in the direction of the left atrium from the mitral valve at contraction. The mitral valve regurgitation bundle may be located in a central or eccentric area. Cine MRI also directly displays the shape, size, thickness, and activity of the valve and sometimes can directly detect the valve dropping into the left atrium. On the heart short-axis perpendicular to the ventricular septum, cine MRI measures the enlarged mitral annulus diameter. MRI can be utilized with many methods to measure regurgitation when the mitral valve is not completely closed, such as the semiquantitative method, blood measuring quantitative method, and MRI volume measuring quantitative method. When assessing the shape and function of the left ventricle, the MRI volume measuring method is the gold standard for measuring ventricular volume, stroke volume, and blood ejection fractional order myocardial mass. Additionally, when judging incomplete closure of the mitral valve due to ischemic heart disease, MRI heart muscle perfusion can be adopted to identify myocardial ischemia and the scope and degree of the infarct area to assess viable myocardium.

3. Mitral Valve Stenosis Accompanied by Regurgitation

When both a stenosis and regurgitation coexist, the above imaging expressions will all appear, and with quickened disease development, the symptoms will develop early, such as augmentation of the atria and ventricles, an increase in the RVESV, a decrease in the LVEDV, RVSV, and RVEF, and RVEDV, as well as and RV-mass augmentation or shrinking.

CONCLUSION

Both CT and MRI can clearly show the shape and structure of the mitral valve. CT has advantages of short imaging time, high time and space resolution, good repetition, ability to detect calcified lesions, and the capability of measuring relevant blood dynamic parameters semiquantitatively, whereas MRI detects the blood signal changes that occur in valvular heart diseases well, can be used to quantitatively measure the degree of valve stenosis or regurgitation volume, and can accurately measure functional changes in the left ventricle. These imaging methods offer enough accurate information for clinicians when assessing mitral valve lesions and supplement the shortcomings of ultrasonic cardiogram examinations.

REFERENCES

[1] Alpert J.S. et al, as the editor-in-chief, Guo Jihong, translator, *Cardiac valvular disease*, third edition, Beijing Science Press, 2003:1-164.

[2] Rahimtoola SH, Frye RL. Valvular heart disease. *Circulation* 2000;102:IV-24 –IV-33.

[3] Wang Jiyao, editor-in-chief, Internal Medicine, first edition, Beijing People's Health Press, 2005:299-310

[4] Sims JM, Miracle VA. An overview of mitral valve prolapse. *Dimens Crit Care Nurs* 2007;26 (4):145-149.

[5] Cawley PJ, Maki JH, Otto CM. Cardiovascular magnetic resonance imaging for valvular heart disease technique and validation. *Circulation* 2009;119:468-478.

[6] Alkadhi H, Bettex D, Wildermuth S, et al. Dynamic cine imaging of the mitral valve with 16-MDCT: a feasibility study. *AJR* 2005; 185:636–646.

[7] Wood P. An appreciation of mitral stenosis part I clinical features. *Br Med J* 1954;1:1051.

[8] Essop MR, Nkomo VT. Rheumatic and nonrheumatic valvular heart disease epidemiology, management, and prevention in Africa. *Circulation* 2005;112:3584-3591.

[9] Li Gandi, editor-in-chief, *Pathology,* first edition, Beijing People's Health Press, 2001:174-182

[10] McKusick VA. Cardiovascular sound in: health and disease. *Baltimore, Md: Williams & Wilkins* 1958:129.

[11] Barlow JB, Pocock WA, Marchand P, et al. The significance of late systolic murmurs. *Am Heart J* 1963;66:443– 452.

[12] Criley JM, Lewis KB, Humphries JO, et al. Prolapse of the mitral valve:clinical and cine-angiographic findings. *Br Heart J* 1966;28:488–496.

[13] Edler I, Hertz CH. The use of ultrasonic reflectoscope for the continuous recording of the movements of heart walls. *Kungliga Fysiografiska Sallskapets i Lund Forhandlingar* 1954;24:1–19.

[14] Salehian O, Chan KL. Impact of three-dimensional echocardiography in valvular heart disease. *Current Opinion in Cardiology* 2005, 20:122-126.

[15] Zamorano J, Alberto de Agustı´n J. Three-dimensional echocardiography for assessment of mitral valve stenosis. *Current Opinion in Cardiology* 2009,24:000–000.

[16] Messika-Zeitoun D, Brochet E, Holmin C, et al. Three-dimensional evaluation of the mitral valve area and commissural opening before and after percutaneous mitral commissurotomy in patients with mitral stenosis. *Eur Heart J* 2007 Jan;28 (1):72-9.

[17] Chen JJ, Manning MA, Frazier AA, Jeudy J, White CS. CT angiography of the cardiac valves: normal, diseased, and postoperative appearances. *Radiographics* 2009 Sep-Oct;29 (5):1393-412.

[18] Konen E, Goitein O, Feinberg MS, et al. The role of ECG-gated MDCT in the evaluation of aortic and mitral mechanical valves: initial experience. *AJR* 2008; 191:26–31.

[19] Savino G, Zwerner P, Herzog C, et al. CT of cardiac function. *J Thorac Imaging* 2007;22:86–100.

[20] Sugeng L, Mor-Avi V, Weinert L, et al. Quantitative assessment of left ventricular size and function: side-by-side comparison of real-time three-dimensional echocardiography and computed tomography with magnetic resonance reference. *Circulation* 2006; 114: 654-661.

[21] Lawrence MB. CT of valvular heart disease. *Int J Cardiovasc Imag* 2005; 21:105-113.

[22] Ryan R, Abbara S, Colen RR, et al. Cardiac valve disease: spectrum of findings on cardiac 64-MDCT. *AJR* 2008; 190:W294–W303.

[23] Mahnken AH, Mühlenbruch G, Das M, et al. MDCT detection of mitral valve calcification: prevalence and clinical relevance compared with echocardiography. *AJR* 2007; 188:1264–1269.

[24] Donnino R, Jacobs JE, Doshi JV, et al. Dual-source versus single-source cardiac CT angiography: comparision of diagnostic image quality. *AJR* 2009;192:1051-1056.

[25] Rerkpattanapipat P, Mazur W, Link KM, Hundley WG. Assessment of cardiac function with MR imaging. *Magn Reson Imaging Clin N Am* 2003;11:67–80.

[26] Tandri H, Castillo E, Ferrari VA, et al. Magnetic resonance imaging of arrhythmogenic right ventricular dysplasia sensitivity, specificity, and observer variability of fat detection versus functional analysis of the right ventricle. *JACC* 2006; 48: 2277-2284

[27] Rozenshtein A, Boxt LM. Computed tomography and magnetic resonance imaging of patients with valvular heart disease. *Journal of Thoracic Imaging* 2000.15:252–264.

[28] Deng W, Yang ZG, Peng LQ, et al, Morphological and dynamic features of normal mitral valve evaluated by dual-source computed tomography. *Int J Cardiol.* 2010;145 (3):633-6.

[29] Zoghbi WA, Enriquez-Sarano M, Foster E, et al. Recommendations for evaluation of the severity of native valvular regurgitation with two-dimensional and doppler echocardiography.*J Am Soc Echocardiogr* 2003;16:777–802.

[30] Guo YK, Gao HL, Zhang XC, et al. Accuracy and reproducibility of assessing right ventricular function with 64-section multi-detector row CT: comparison with magnetic resonance imaging. *Int J Cardiol.* 2010;139 (3):254-62.

[31] Guo YK, Yang ZG, Ning G, et al. Isolated mitral regurgitation: quantitative assessment with 64-section multidetector CT—comparison with MR imaging and echocardiography. *Radiology* 2009;252 (2):369-76.

[32] Guo YK, Yang ZG, Ning G, et al. Sixty-four-slice multidetector computed tomography for preoperative evaluation of left ventricular function and mass in patients with mitral regurgitation: comparison with magnetic resonance imaging and echocardiography. *Eur Radiol* 2009;19 (9):2107-16.

In: Mitral Valve Disease
Editor: Richard R. Heuser
ISBN: 978-1-61942-309-1

Chapter 6

PERCUTANEOUS MITRAL VALVE REPAIR: STATE OF THE ART

Richard R. Heuser **[1]** ***and Shishir Murarka*** **[2]**
[1]St. Luke's Medical Center, Phoenix, Arizona, US
University of Arizona, College of Medicine, Tucson, Arizona, US
[2]Banner Estrella Medical Center, Phoenix, Arizona, US

INTRODUCTION

About 2% of the population in the United States suffers from 'significant' mitral regurgitation (MR) [1]. Surgery is indicated for symptomatic patients or asymptomatic patients with decreased left ventricular ejection fraction [2]. Many patients who have MR have considerable comorbidities for high risk surgery, and less invasive approach may be beneficial for these patients. Percutaneous treatment for valvular diseases is attractive because it provides a less traumatic alternative avoiding sternotomy and cardio-pulmonary bypass, which means lesser complications and shorter hospital stay. Hence, the concept of percutaneous repair is encouraging and merits attention. An ideal Mitral valve (MV) repair should achieve normal coaptation of the leaflets and maintain leaflet mobility, without injuring the adjacent structures. During the last decade, a considerable progress has been made in the development of transcatheter devices and techniques to treat MR. Some percutaneous techniques for treatment of MR utilize the existing surgical principles, while some are based on novel concepts. These techniques are in various stages of development, ranging from pre-clinical investigation phase to early phase of clinical application. These techniques could be broadly grouped based on the target areas of treatment: annuloplasty (indirect and direct), leaflet repair, and chamber remodeling.

ANNULOPLASTY

Surgical annuloplasty is considered the main modality of treatment patients with functional MR. Functional MR results from increase in the septal-lateral or antero-posterior annular diameter due to ischemic or dilated cardiomyopathy. This is targeted in surgical repair by the use of an undersized complete and rigid annuloplasty ring anchored in the fibrous trigone. This same principle of increasing the leaflet coaptation by reducing the septal – lateral annular diameter forms the basis of percutaneous mitral valve repair. This can be achieved by either placing a device in the coronary sinus (indirect annuloplasty) or direct implantation of device into the mitral annulus (direct annuloplasty).

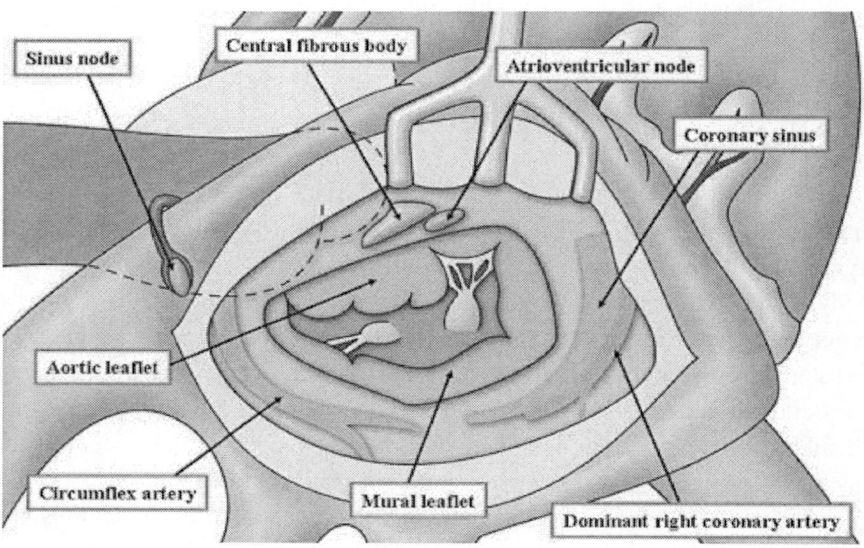

Figure 1. Anatomical Structures Surrounding the Left Atrioventricular Junction. Relationships of the mitral valve as seen by the surgeon operating through the roof of the left atrium.

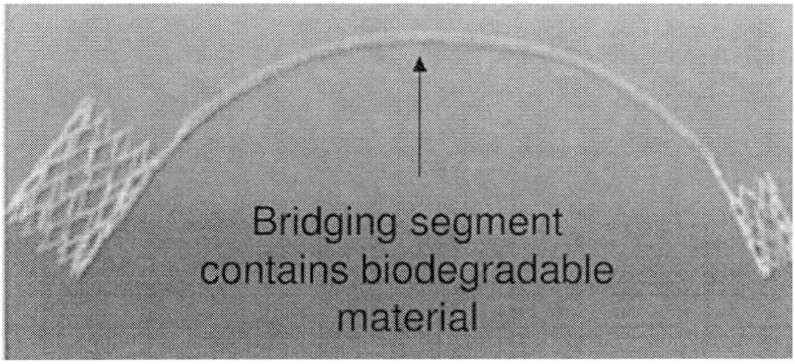

Figure 2. The MONARC System.
The support frame is constructed of nitinol. Intervening between the proximal and distal stent anchors is a spring-like bridging segment with memory characteristics and biodegradable material.

Indirect Annuloplasty

Indirect annuloplasty capitalizes on the anatomical proximity of coronary sinus to mitral annulus (Figure 1). The coronary sinus courses in the atrioventricular groove in direct proximity of the posterior mitral annulus and encircles about two-thirds of the mitral annulus. Placement of an annuloplasty device in the coronary sinus can push against the posterior portion of mitral annulus, therefore, alter MV geometry and reduce the annulus diameter. Coronary sinus can be easily accessed through the Internal Jugular Vein or Subclavian Vein. Several devices are in clinical testing phase – the Monarc device (Edwards Lifesciences, Irvine, CA), the Carillon Mitral Contour System (Cardiac Dimensions Inc, Kirkland, WA), and the PTMA device (Viacor Inc, Wilmington, MA).

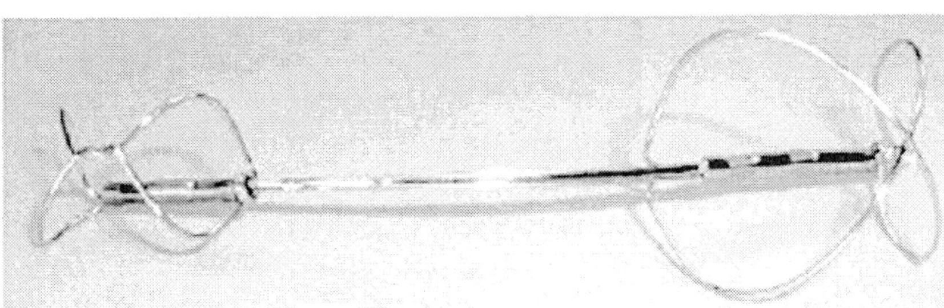

Figure 3. The CARILLON Mitral Contour System.

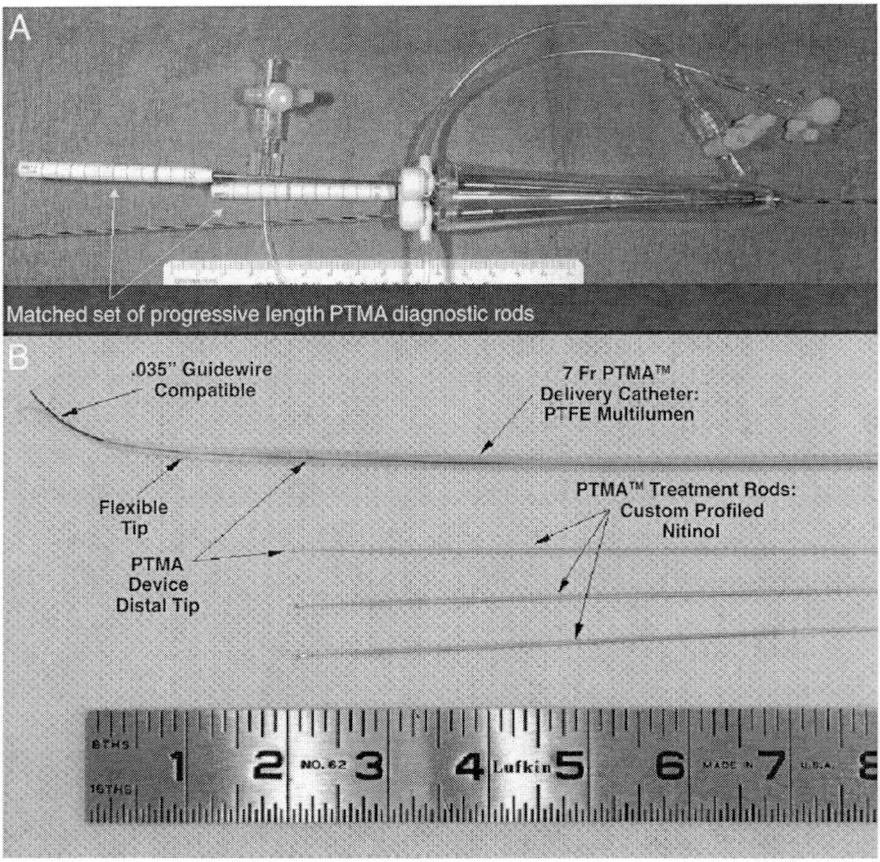

Figure 4. The PTMA Device.

The Monarc device (Edwards Lifesciences, Irvine, CA) consists of two self-expanding nitinol stents anchors separated by an extended spring bridge element (Figure 2). The distal stent is delivered in the anterior interventricular vein, a tributary of the great cardiac vein and the proximal stent is placed in the coronary sinus. The spaces of the spring are kept open by biodegradable material filling these spaces. The bioabsorbable material degrades over several weeks; the spring shortens and applies tension on the coronary sinus and the adjacent annulus. The clinical efficacy of this device is not evident for at least a few weeks after implantation till the spring shortens. Among the first five reported patients, the bridge fractured in three, and reduction in MR was seen in three of the four patients [3]. The device was subsequently redesigned to avoid separations. In a recently published results from the EVOLUTION phase I study, the MONARC device was implanted in 59 of 72 patients (82%) with MR grade ≥ 2 were enrolled at 8 participating centers in 4 countries. At 12 months, a reduction in MR by ≥ 1 grade was observed in 50.0% of 22 implanted patients with matched echocardiograms and in 85.7% of 7 patients with baseline MR grade ≥ 3 [4]. The study concluded that implantation of the MONARC device in the coronary sinus is feasible and may reduce MR. However, coronary artery compression may occur in patients in whom the great cardiac vein passes over a coronary artery, necessitating strategies to avoid this occurrence.

The Carillon Mitral Contour System (Cardiac Dimensions Inc, Kirkland, WA) uses a nitinol wire made into a proximal and distal anchor connected by a nitinol bridge (Figure 3). The distal anchor is deployed in the great cardiac vein. Manual Tension is applied to the connecting wire that is progressively shortened until an appropriate reduction in mitral regurgitation is achieved. The proximal anchor is then released in the coronary sinus. The device was redesigned (CARILLON XE) to address the problems with anchoring seen in first generation devices [5]. The AMADEUS trial enrolled 48 patients; device implantation was successful in 30 patients. At 6 months, the degree of functional MR reduction among 5 different quantitative echocardiographic measures ranged from 22% to 32%. Significant improvement in six-minute walk distance and the quality of life was noted as well [6].

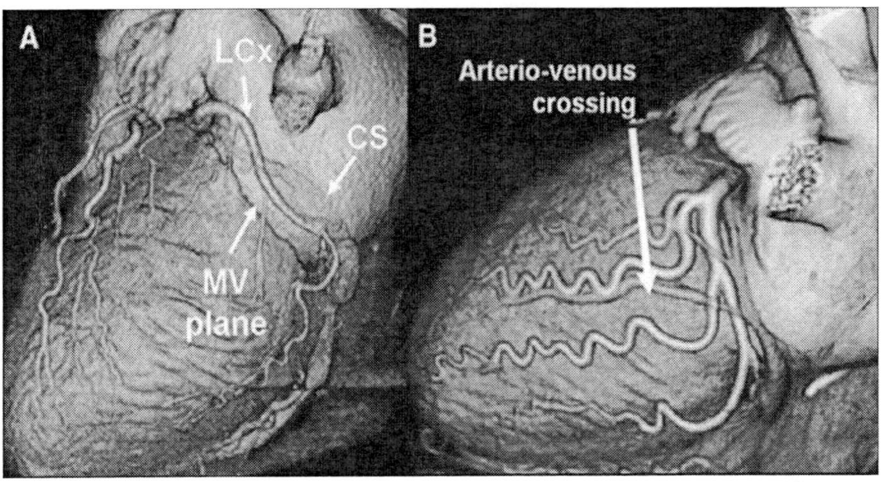

Figure 5. Computed tomography images showing relationship between the plane of the mitral valve (MV), the left circumflex coronary artery (LCx) and the coronary sinus (CS).

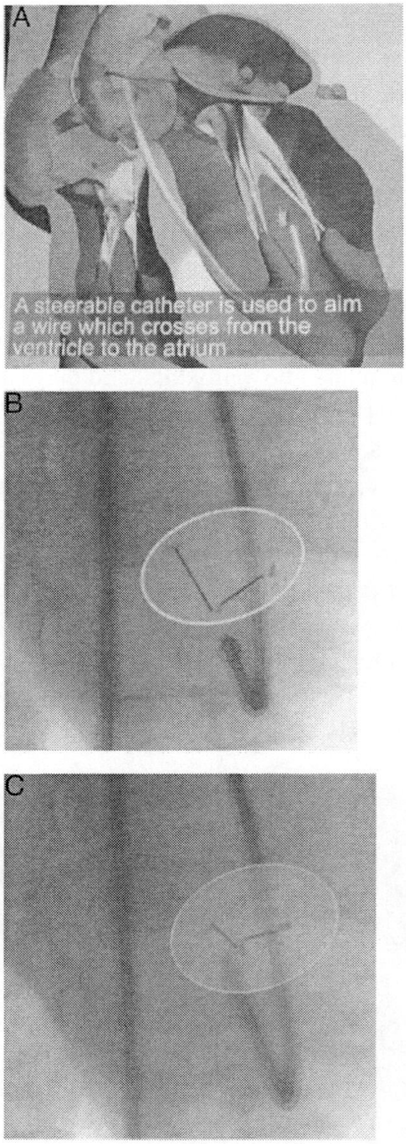

Figure 6. The Mitralign System (A) Illustration depicting the therapy catheter with a deflectable end inserted retrograde across the aortic valve into the left ventricle and positioned in a subvalvar mitral position. (B and C) Tethering and tension on the system brings the anchors in closer proximity, resulting in a reduction in the septal-lateral dimension of the mitral annulus.

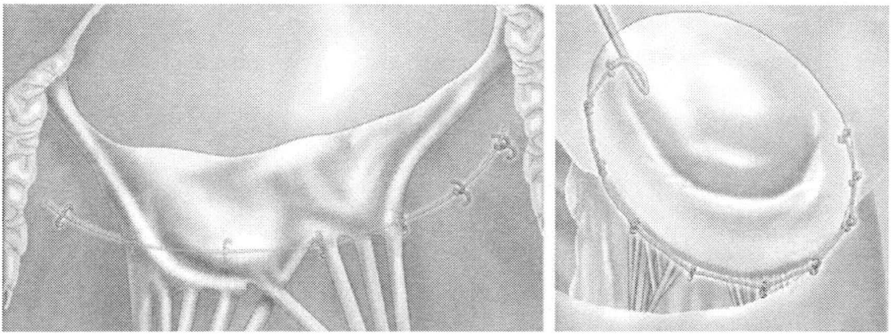

Figure 7. The Guided Delivery Systems Accucinch device is delivered through retrograde catheterization of the left ventricle. (Left) Anchors are placed in the posterior mitral annulus and (right) connected with a "drawstring" to cinch the annular circumference. Figure illustration by Craig Skaggs.

The PTMA device (Viacor Inc, Wilmington, MA) uses nitinol rods of varying length and stiffness, delivered via a catheter to the coronary sinus via the subclavian route (Figure 4). Nitinol rods are placed into the three lumens of the delivery catheter so that pressure can be applied to the posterior annulus at the P2 segment to compress the septal-lateral annulus dimension. Rod stiffness can be changed until some diminution in MR is achieved. The rod can be exchanged at a future time if additional stiffness is needed, or can be removed if there are any issues with the device. In contrast to other coronary sinus devices encircling and constricting the mitral annulus, the PTMA method 'compresses' the septal lateral dimension. Preliminary human experience with this device has shown reduction in mitral annular dimension that persisted over several months [7].

Coronary sinus approach is simple and can be used to deliver a device in beating heart. There are, however, several limitations to this approach. This technique utilizes the proximity of coronary sinus to the mitral annulus; however, the anatomic relationship of the sinus to the mitral annulus is variable [8, 9]. The gap between them measures 5-8mm in most patients that may widen in patients with severe MR. This may affect the efficacy of the procedure. The left circumflex coronary artery or one of its branches frequently cross under the coronary sinus (Figure 5). This can compress the circumflex artery and result in myocardial infarction [10]. This was observed in initial trials with the coronary sinus devices. Thus evaluation of coronary arteries, and relationship between coronary sinus, mitral annulus and coronary arteries is essential before the procedure. Other potential areas for complications are long-term erosion or thrombosis of the coronary sinus, device fracture from the mechanical stresses of the coronary sinus or presence of other devices in the coronary sinus that may preclude placement of these devices.

Direct Annuloplasty

This technique aims at device mediated mitral annulus reshaping using a direct approach rather than using coronary sinus. This overcomes some of the limitations encountered in coronary sinus techniques.

The Mitralign Percutaneous Annuloplasty System (Mitralign, Tewksbury, MA) approaches the posterior mitral annulus via the left ventricle (Figure 6). A guide catheter is passed via the Femoral artery across the aortic valve into the left ventricle and is placed directly beneath the mid-posterior mitral leaflet. A specially designed catheter with two tips (Bident) is used to place two to four anchors through the posterior annulus. The mitral annulus is penetrated using radiofrequency wires and access to the left atrium is achieved. 2 pairs of surgical pledgets are delivered over the wires and anchored across the posterior mitral annulus from the left atrium to the left ventricle. The surgical pledgets are then tethered and put into tension to decrease the annulus circumference. This device has been successfully used in first –in- man studies [11].

The Accucinch Annuloplasty System (Guided Delivery Systems, Inc, Santa Clara, CA) uses nine to 12 nitinol anchors that can be placed from the anterior to the posterior commisures once access to the left ventricle is achieved using the retrograde femoral artery approach (Figure 7). These anchors are then connected with a tether or cord that draws the anchors together. This system has been successfully used in first –in- man studies as well [11].

The Quantum Cor System (Quantum Cor Inc, Lake Forest, CA) utilizes the application of radiofrequency energy to shrink the mitral annulus. The mitral annuli is an area dense in collagen and heat has been shown shrink collagen. Using this principle, favorable results were obtained in sheep model (Figure 8). The QuantumCor system uses a probe that incorporates seven electrodes (~1.5 mm × 2 mm) and is malleable and conforms to the annulus shape. Delivery of radiofrequency energy to electrodes was computer controlled by maximum temperatures sensed by adjacent thermocouples. The annuli were treated circumferentially (from the posterior annulus) using temperatures set at 65 °C. The entire posterior annulus was treated from commissure to commissure in 1–2-cm segments. At 180 days, the treatment animals showed significant reduction in the antero-posterior diameter of the mitral annulus with mean annular reduction of 26.4%. This system is in pre-clinical phase and human studies are yet to be carried out [12].

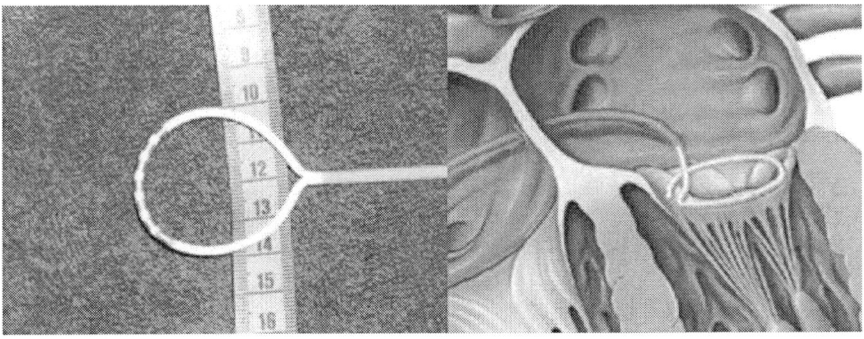

Figure 8. QuantumCor Device. The QuantumCor device (QuantumCor, Lake Forest, California) (left) and device applied to the mitral annulus via the transseptal approach (right).

Leaflet Repair

The leaflet repair simulates the surgical edge to edge' repair or double orifice repair pioneered by Alfieri [13]. The edge-to-edge repair reduces MR by bringing together the middle of the anterior and posterior mitral leaflets or creating a double orifice, thereby effectively eliminating some of the redundant tissue and reducing MR.

The MitraClip system (Evalve, Menlo Park, CA) utilizes a clip that engages the anterior and posterior leaflets of the mitral valve (figure 9). The MitraClip system uses a guide catheter, a clip delivery system and an implantable tip. The guide catheter is 24 F proximally, 22 F at the atrial septum and is delivered over a tapered dilator. The clip delivery system has MitraClip attached to its distal end. The MitraClip device is a 4mm wide cobalt chromium implant with 2 arms. The two arms have an opened span of about 2 cm when opened in the grasping position. The arms are opened and closed by a mechanism on the delivery catheter handle. There are 2 grippers on the inner portion of the clip to secure the leaflets. The procedure is performed under general anesthesia with guidance from echocardiography and fluoroscopy. The guide is delivered to the left atrium via the transseptal route using the femoral vein access. The clip delivery system is introduced into the guide catheter and is advanced and manipulated so that the clip is at the center of the mitral orifice. The clip is then opened and advanced into the left ventricle below the mitral leaflets. The clip is then retracted until the mitral leaflets are captured and then closed to coapt the mitral leaflets (figure 10). The degree of MR can be assessed using Doppler echocardiography, and if needed the clip can be opened and closed several times or a second clip may be placed to obtain adequate results.

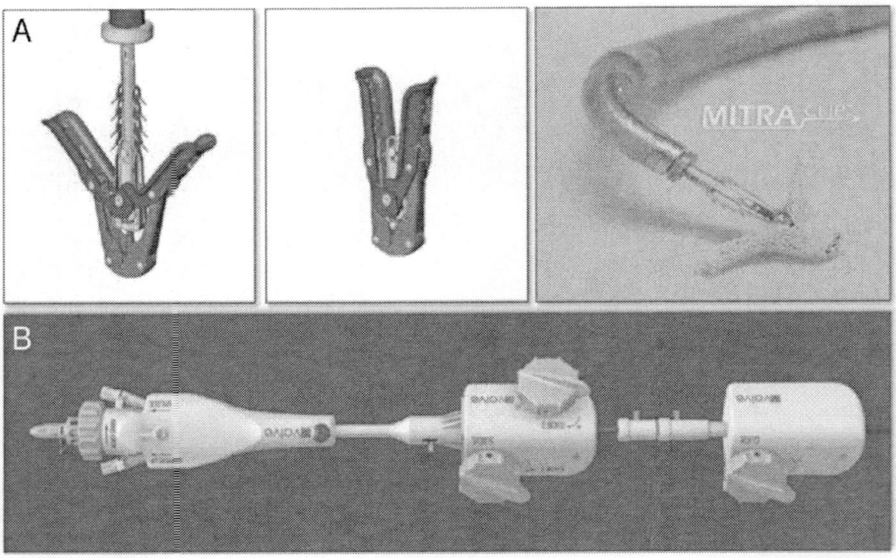

Figure 9. The Evalve MitraClip.
(A) The Evalve MitraClip. The clip arms are open (left) when the device is passed across the mitral leaflets from the left atrium into the left ventricle. The gripper is the barbed piece seen in the upper left panel, parallel to the shaft of the delivery system. When the leaflets are grasped, the gripper helps to fix the leaflets within the clip arms (middle). The clip is covered with polyester fabric (right). (B) The steering knobs are shown on the right-hand side of the device for maneuvering the clip within the left atrial cavity. At the far left of the picture is the knob that is used to open and close the clip, and the release mechanism.

The EVEREST (Endovascular Valve Edge to Edge Repair Study) was a prospective multicenter single arm study to evaluate the feasibility, safety and efficacy of this system in patients that had 3-4+ MR using the AHA/ACC (American Heart Association/. American College of Cardiology) guidelines. Acute procedural success was achieved in 74% of the patients and 64 % were discharged with MR ≤ 1+. Nine percent patients had major adverse even, including 1 non-procedural death [14]. The EVEREST II Trial is a multicenter randomized controlled trial to evaluate the benefits and risks of the MitraClip device compared with open mitral valve surgery (control) in patients with moderate or severe MR. Using a 2:1 randomization ratio, the trial enrolled 186 MitraClip-treated subjects and 93 control subjects. The results of the trial were presented at ACC 2010. The MitraClip system demonstrated a superior safety profile compared to surgical repair or replacement (9.6% of MitraClip patients and 57% of surgery patients had an major adverse event). In the primary effectiveness endpoint, the MitraClip device was noninferior to surgery at 1 year (clinical success rate of 72.4% for MitraClip patients with successful initial treatment compared to a clinical success rate of 87.8% for surgery patients) [15].

The Mobius device (Edward Life Sciences, Irving, CA) used suture based system [16] instead of clip, however the program has been terminated because of technical difficulties and disappointing results in humans.

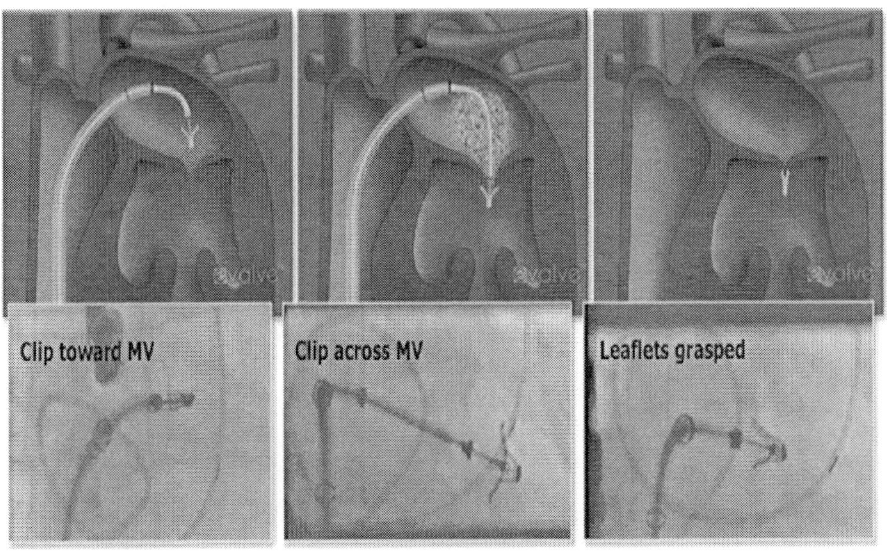

Figure 10. Basic Steps of the Evalve MitraClip Clip Procedure (Top) The left panel shows the clip being steered through the left atrium toward the center of the mitral orifice. The middle panel illustrates the device across the mitral valve (MV) with the clip arms open, before the clip has been pulled back to grasp the mitral leaflets. The right panel shows, in the cartoon, the clip has been released. (Bottom) In the fluoroscopic figure, the leaflets have been grasped and clipped closed partially, before full closure and release of the clip.

Chamber Remodeling

The Percutaneous Septal Sinus Shortening System (PS3 System, Ample Medical, Foster City, CA) uses a bridge system to connect anchor in the coronary sinus to the anchor in the interatrial septum. Tension applied on the bridge reduces the septal-lateral dimensions and reduces MR [17]. Using animal model, the investigators found that device implantation resulted in acute and chronic MR reduction [18]. This technique had excellent safety with reductions in MR in first in man [19], however further device development has been abandoned.

The iCoapsys system (Myocor, Apple Grove, Minnesota) is based on the surgically placed iCoapsys system that was initially placed at the time of coronary artery bypass grafting in patients with ischemic MR [20]. Under fluoroscopic and echocardiography guidance, intrapericardial anchoring devices are placed on the epicardial left ventricular anterior and posterior surfaces and connected by a transventricular tethering suture (figure 11). Left ventricular geometry can be changed by applying tension to the suture. This device remodels the left ventricular chamber and compresses the mitral annular septo posterior dimension. Studies have demonstrated feasibility of the percutaneous iCoapsys procedure in an ovine model [21]; unfortunately, this device development has been discontinued at the current time because of financial limitations.

Other Techniques

Chordal Implantation

Percutaneous chordal procedures are being developed based on the concept of chordal repair, implantation, or removal during surgical mitral valve repair. The DS1000 device, developed to deploy Neochordae (Neochord, Minnetonka, Minnesota) to the mitral leaflet with subsequent anchorage to the apex of the left ventricle, has shown encouraging results and is undergoing initial clinical investigation [22].

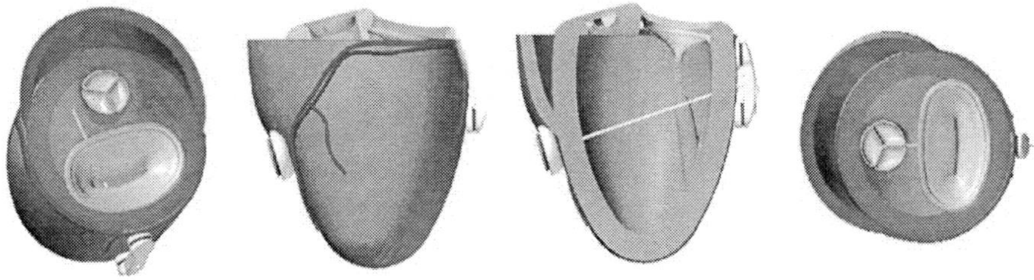

Figure 11. The Coapsys system. The tether places tension on the septal-lateral dimension of the mitral valve and also remodels the basal left ventricle with reorientation of the papillary muscles.

Mitral Valve Replacement

Several companies are developing percutaneous or minimally invasive mitral valve replacement. The Endovalve-Hermann prosthesis (Endovalve, Princeton, New Jersey) is a mitral valve replacement system (23) initially designed for minimally invasive procedure. The device is a foldable nitinol structure that attaches to the native valve (Figure 12). The system is delivered into the left atrium via right minithoracotomy, with a specially designed delivery device and removable cables that allow contraction, repositioning and release. As opposed to the aortic valve, the mitral devices will need to be much larger, and will not be implanted using radial force as fixation method since the valve is usually not calcified in case of MR, and because radial expansion of the valve would induce aortic valve deformations and outflow tract obstruction. CardiAQ Valve (Winchester, Massachusetts) is developing a novel percutaneous solution that doesn't use a radial force to attach the artificial valve (Figure13).

CONCLUSION

Percutaneous mitral valve treatment is a rapidly emerging. Many different devices are in the pipeline for optimal percutaneous treatment of MR. The results of from the EVEREST II trial, the only randomized controlled trial so far, are encouraging. The other devices that are being developed have interesting concepts and further clinical experience will reveal their strengths and weaknesses. As with most cardiovascular procedures, the impetus for developing effective percutaneous mitral valve repair will continue to strenghten as it hold a great promise for better outcomes and for those patients who cannot undergo surgical treatment.

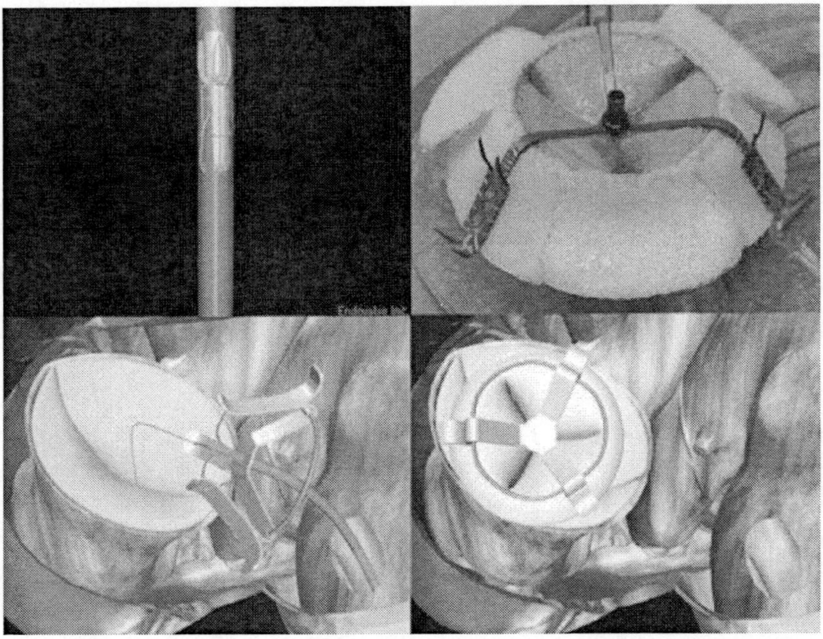

Figure 12. Endovalve-Herrmann Prosthesis.
The Endovalve-Herrmann prosthesis (top right), loaded in the delivery sheath (top left), and sequence of implantation (bottom left and right).

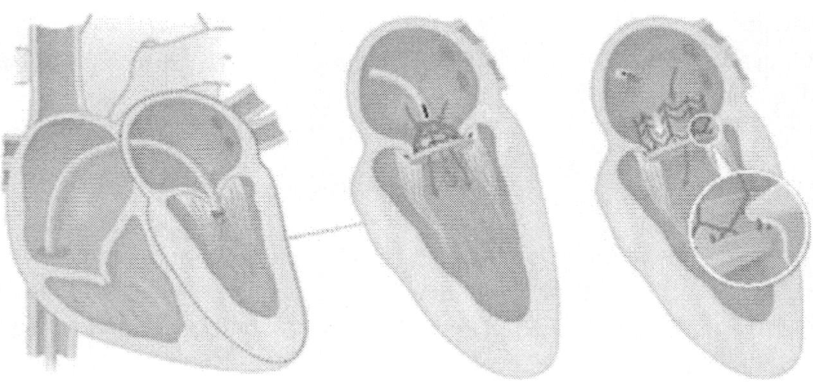

Figure 13. CardiAQ Prosthesis.
The CardiAQ (CardiAQ Valve Technologies, Inc., Winchester, Massachusetts). prosthesis; this device is delivered transseptally (left) and locks onto the inferior (middle) and superior (right) surfaces of the mitral annulus.

REFERENCES

[1] Jones EC, Devereux RB, Roman MJ, et al: Prevalence and correlates of mitral regurgitation in a population-based sample (the Strong Heart study). *Am J Cardiol.* 2001, 87: 298-304.

[2] Bonow RO, Carabello BA, Chatterjee K, et al: 2006 Writing Committee Members; American College of Cardiology/American Heart Association Task Force. 2008 Focused update incorporated into the ACC/AHA 2006 guidelines for the management of patients with valvular heart disease: a report of the American College of Cardiology/American Heart Association Task Force on Practice Guidelines (Writing Committee to Revise the 1998 Guidelines for the Management of Patients With Valvular Heart Disease). *Circulation.* 2008, 118: e523-e661.

[3] Webb JG, Harnek J, Munt BI, Kimblad PO, Chandavimo M, Thompson CR, Mayo JR, Solem JO. Percutaneous transvenous mitral annuloplasty: initial human experience with device implantation in the coronary sinus. *Circulation.* 2006; 113: 851–855.

[4] Harnek J, Webb JG, Kuck KH, Tschope C, Vahanian A, Buller CE, James SK, Tiefenbacher CP, Stone GW. Transcatheter implantation of the MONARC coronary sinus device for mitral regurgitation: 1-year results from the EVOLUTION phase I study (Clinical Evaluation of the Edwards Lifesciences Percutaneous Mitral Annuloplasty System for the Treatment of Mitral Regurgitation). *JACC Cardiovasc Interv.* 2011 Jan;4 (1):115-22

[5] Duffy SJ, Federman J, Farrington C, Reuter DG, Richardson M, Kaye DM. Feasibility and short-term efficacy of percutaneous mitral annular reduction for the therapy of functional mitral regurgitation in patients with heart failure. *Catheter Cardiovasc Interv.* 2006; 68: 205–210.

[6] Schofer J, Siminiak T, Haude M, Herrman JP, Vainer J, Wu JC, Levy WC, Mauri L, Feldman T, Kwong RY, Kaye DM, Duffy SJ, Tübler T, Degen H, Brandt MC, Van Bibber R, Goldberg S, Reuter DG, Hoppe UC. Percutaneous mitral annuloplasty for functional mitral regurgitation: results of the CARILLON Mitral Annuloplasty Device European Union Study. *Circulation.* 2009 Jul 28;120 (4):326-33

[7] Sack S, Kahlert P, Bilodeau L, Pièrard LA, Lancellotti P, Legrand V, Bartunek J, Vanderheyden M, Hoffmann R, Schauerte P, Shiota T, Marks DS, Erbel R, Ellis SG. Percutaneous transvenous mitral annuloplasty: initial human experience with a novel coronary sinus implant device. *Circ Cardiovasc Interv.* 2009 Aug;2 (4):277-84.

[8] Maselli D, Guarracino F, Chiaramonti F, Mangia F, Borelli G, Minzioni G. Percutaneous mitral annuloplasty: an anatomic study of human coronary sinus and its relation with mitral valve annulus and coronary arteries. *Circulation.* 2006; 114: 377–380.

[9] Lansac E, Di Centa I, Al Attar N, Messika-Zeitoun D, Raffoul R, Vahanian A, Nataf P. Percutaneous mitral annuloplasty through the coronary sinus: an anatomic point of view. *J Thorac Cardiovasc Surg.* 2008; 135: 376–381.

[10] Goldberg SL, Van Bibber R, Schofer J, Ebner A, Siminiak T, Hoppe UC, Haude M, Herrman J-PR, Duffy SJ, Reuter D, Kaye DM. The frequency of coronary artery compression and management using a removable mitral annuloplasty device in the coronary sinus. *J Am Coll Cardiol.* 2008; 51 (10 Suppl B): 28.

[11] Feldman T, Ciligiroglu M. Percutaneous leaflet repair and annuloplasty for mitral regurgitation. *J Am Coll Cardiol.* 2011;57:529-37.

[12] Heuser RR, Witzel T, Dickens D, Takeda PA. Percutaneous treatment for mitral regurgitation: the QuantumCor system. *J Interv Cardiol.* 2008; 21: 178–182.

[13] Maisano F, Torracca L, Oppizzi M, Stefano PL, D'Addario G, La Canna G, Zogno M, Alfieri O. The edge-to-edge technique: a simplified method to correct mitral insufficiency. *Eur J Cardiothorac Surg.* 1998; 13: 240–246.

[14] Feldman T, Kar S, Rinaldi M, Fail P, Hermiller J, Smalling R, Whitlow PL, Gray W, Low R, Herrmann HC, Lim S, Foster E, Glower D; EVEREST Investigators. Percutaneous mitral repair with the MitraClip system: safety and midterm durability in the initial EVEREST (Endovascular Valve Edge-to-Edge REpair Study) cohort. *J Am Coll Cardiol.* 2009 Aug 18;54 (8):686-94.

[15] *EVEREST II Data Presented at ACC for Abbott Vascular's MitraClip System.* http://bmctoday.net/citoday/2010/02/article.asp?f=everest-ii-data-presented-at-acc-for-abbott-vasculars-mitraclip-system. Accessed March 21,2011.

[16] Naqvi TZ, Buchbinder M, Zarbatany D, Webb J, Logan J, Molloy M, Balke G, Tieu T, Ainsworth R, Alfieri O, Maisano F. Edge-to-edge repair utilizing a percutaneous suture device in an animal model. *Cathet Cardiovasc Interv.* 2007; 69: 525–531.

[17] Rogers JH, Macoviak JA, Rahdert DA, Takeda PA, Palacios IF, Low RI. Percutaneous septal shortening. A novel procedure for the treatment of functional mitral regurgitation. *Circulation.* 2006; 113: 2329–2334.

[18] Rogers JH, Rahdert DA, Caputo GR, Takeda PA, Palacios IF, Tio FO, Taylor EA, Low RI. Long-term safety and durability of percutaneous septal sinus shortening (the PS3 system TM) in an ovine model. *Catheter Cardiovasc Interv.* 2009; 73: 540–548.

[19] Palacios IF, Condado JA, Brandi S, Rodriquez V, Bosch F, Silva G, Low RI, Rogers JH. Safety and feasibility of acute percutaneous septal sinus shortening: first-in-human experience. *Cathet Cardiovasc Interv.* 2007; 69: 513–518.

[20] Grossi EA, Saunders PC, Woo YJ, Gangahar DM, Laschinger JC, Kress DC, Caskey MP, Schwartz CF, Wudel J. Intraoperative effects of the Coapsys annuloplasty system in a randomized evaluation (RESTOR-MV) of functional ischemic mitral regurgitation. *Ann Thorac Surg.* 2005; 80: 1706–1711.

[21] Pedersen WR, Block P, Leon M, Kramer P, Kapadia S, Babaliaros V, Susheel K, Tuzcu ME, Feldman T. iCoapsys mitral valve repair system: percutaneous implantation in an animal model. *Catheter Cardiovasc Interv.* 2008; 72: 125–131

[22] Seeburger J, Borger MA Mohr FW. Transcatheter mitral valve repair: a high mountain to climb. *Eur Heart J Suppl* (2010) 12 (suppl E): E46-E51.

[23] Chiam PT, Ruiz CE. Percutaneous transcatheter mitral valve repair: a classification of the technology. *JACC Cardiovasc Interv.* 2011 Jan;4 (1):1-13.

INDEX

C

D

E

F

G

H

I

N

O

P

Q

R

S

T

U

V

W

Y